COVET

THE "DISRESPECTFUL" HEALTH AND WELLNESS JOURNAL

Sagashus T. Levingston PhD

VOLUME ONE

LITTLE CREEK PRESS®
AND BOOK DESIGN
MINERAL POINT, WISCONSIN

Copyright © 2022 Sagashus T. Levingston PhD

Little Creek Press®
A Division of Kristin Mitchell Design, Inc.
5341 Sunny Ridge Road
Mineral Point, Wisconsin 53565

Book Design and Project Coordination:
Little Creek Press and Book Design

First printing
March 2022

All rights reserved

No part of this book may be used or reproduced
in any manner whatsoever without written
permission from the author.

Printed in the United States of America

For more information or to order books
www.infamousmothers.com
www.littlecreekpress.com

ISBN: 978-1-955656-15-3

COVET

Welcome

Welcome to Covet: The Disrespectful Health and Wellness Journal. As the CEO/founder of the Infamous Mothers brand, I am excited you are here.

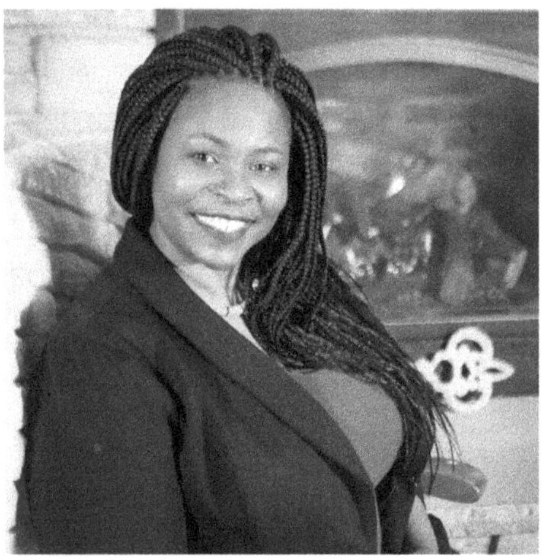

I created this journal as a companion for our Covet fitness program (offered as an amenity to our 3rd Space Virtual Coworking). Its contents are both a compilation of the lessons learned from our members and fitness instructors as well as a response to the needs expressed by them. Equally important, this book is exactly the kind of journal I've been searching for in bookstores and big-box stores but haven't found. Its approach is holistic, focusing on the mind, body, spirit, and emotions. While there is some structure and consistency, there is a lot of flexibility and variety, making your journaling experience as exciting and adventurous as your health and wellness journey itself.

The Infamous Mothers brand has always been about community and bridging gaps. We continue that work with this journal. It marries the analog with the digital, the mind with the body, goals with their whys, and so much more. Bringing together a chorus of voices that include current Covet members, friends of Covet, and experts from the health and fitness industry, I embedded community in its pages so that you will always be reminded that you are part of a movement and a collective. You are not alone, and you will succeed.

Over the past five years, our work has focused on expanding the narrative around Infamous Mothers. That has included helping them conceptualize, build, and grow sustainable businesses. Recently, it has included a focus on wealth generation. We've learned some things in that process. One of the biggest takeaways is this: In a racist, classist, sexist, homophobic world, focusing on wealth building without focusing on the health and wellness of those starting and growing companies and brands undermines our efforts. It is to ignore the impact that microaggressions, discrimination, psychological violence, police brutality, revenue gaps, and so much more, have on the overall health of those in our society who devote a significant part of their lives caring for others, especially mothers who build their mothering practice outside of respectability politics and the status quo. This journal is for them—for us.

We are not martyrs, and we will not trade in our health and wellness as a price for success. We will not collapse at the threshold of our goals. Instead, we will be healthy and happy and whole, two-stepping, twerking, cha-cha sliding, and wining our way across the finish lines of our milestones. That's my vision for two million infamous mothers worldwide. May every one of you reach your milestones and chronicle your journey as part of the legend that is you. May every one of you build your health alongside your wealth. And may each of you be forever Infamous

—Dr. Sagashus

About This Journal

Covet: The "Disrespectful" Health and Wellness Journal is in a class of its own. It invites you to explore multiple aspects of your overall well-being and prompts you to connect your mind, body, emotions, and spirit, asking you to take a systems approach to wellness. It creates space for you to address trauma as a part of your health and wellness trek. And while this journal is inspired by and created for the women in our fitness program, it is for any person who identifies as a badass mom on a health and wellness adventure. This journal was created for anyone looking to be inspired, held accountable, build new habits, establish a mind-body connection, and reach their health and wellness goals. Whether you are new to journaling or are deeply committed to a long-term practice, this book is for you. Most importantly, it recognizes the value of having a safe space away from the worlds (both private and public) that may sometimes make you feel vulnerable or afraid. A world inundated with -isms—racism, classism, sexism, etc.—make it more challenging for us to tend to our health and wellness, as they impose violence, endangering our well-being on every level. This journal (and the workshops, retreats, and fitness classes that accompany it) offer you shelter, protection, and a break from some of those dangers.

Why a Journal?

Research tells us that we are more likely to accomplish our goals if we write them down. But where do you write them? How often do we revisit them? And after you figure this out, what's next? The Covet journal was created to address these and many other questions. For almost one year, members of the Covet fitness program showed up, week after week, for weight training, yoga, and a series of wellness challenges created in conjunction with our pilot wealth program. We noticed that participants who tracked their meals, had a written and clearly stated "why," and a written daily and weekly health and fitness agenda were substantially more successful than members who had not committed their plans in writing. This journal was created to help you create a contract with yourself and help you follow through with it. It's meant to be the storehouse for the vision you will be implementing daily. And it's intended to lovingly keep you on track when your brain wants to forget or go rogue—learning to both respect the process and make peace with the possibility that it may, in fact, respect you as well.

Why THIS Journal?

This journal stands out for many reasons, starting with its name. The word covet means to "yearn to possess or have (something)." For many of us, that word is associated with sin. For example, "thou shalt not covet thy neighbor's goods." But what if what you are yearning for is the best version of yourself? What if becoming your wildest dreams is what you want to possess? This journal is about helping you fulfill your highest vision of yourself.

We call it the "Disrespectful Health and Wellness Journal" for several reasons. For one, it contains cussing. In fact, there is a whole section dedicated to cussing and venting called "Daily Shit." There is space for a "gossip session" with yourself about yourself and your experiences every week called the "Weekly Tea." And daily, you are offered sources of inspiration called "Dirty Words." Most of all, we call it the "disrespectful journal" because that's what the health and wellness journey feels like sometimes.

The scale sometimes feels disrespectful, the healthy choices we have to make feel disrespectful, and the amount of patience and time the journey can sometimes require feels so damned disrespectful. We own all of this so that we can embrace and honor the process and accomplish our goals.

The Infamous Mothers brand has always been communal. The Covet journal is all about sisterhood and collaboration. As you progress through it, expect to encounter the voices of women throughout the nation who are on this walk with you, including mine, Dr. Sagashus Levingston, the founder of Infamous Mothers, LLC, who has—at the time of this writing—lost over 30 pounds and changed my life for the better because of my health and wellness journey with Covet. In addition to my voice, you will encounter the voices of women participating in our pilot cohort. These include fitness instructors who lead our classes, friends of Covet, and diverse experts throughout the fitness industry. Think of your journal writing as a collaboration between you and a sisterhood.

We live in a digital age. And yet, many of our participants struggled to keep up with all the data scattered across the many apps that record their sleep, steps, weight, Wellness Wins (WW) points, etc. They wanted one place to not only give them a collective view but a place to reflect on what those numbers revealed. Covet marries the digital with the analog, offering one place to store all your data as well as a place to create a narrative around it, further deepening that mind-body connection.

Finally, the Covet journal was created to be both beautiful and culturally relevant. Writing can be daunting. To write in a place that feels sterile and scientific can feel violent. We needed to create a journal that felt inviting and humane. It needed to reflect our members' beauty, power, and experiences, as well as their concerns, aspirations, and desires. To this end, we have curated quotes from women we thought could speak to your experiences, included imagery meant to be a reflection of you, and offered writing prompts that will resonate with our community.

How to Use This Journal

Covet is meant to be used daily. How much time you want to spend with it is up to you. We recommend that you kick off your journal writing at one of our Covet retreats. There you will establish your big-picture, 12-week and 4-week goals. We will also work with you on your BIG WHY statement, help you establish your initial numbers (weight, water intake, sleep, etc.), and begin building your health and wellness process. On your own, you will focus on your daily goals. As you might have figured out, goals, why statements and data are very important components to this journal.

It is also important to note that every month has a respective theme: Freedom, Self-Value, and Declare Yourself.

Other important aspects of this book are the Daily Shit sections—the Self-Value Tank is meant to be used as a tool for self-assessment and reflection to help you stay mindful (or develop mindfulness) as you grow on your journey.

Use the Covet journal to keep you inspired, keep you "honest," and keep you accomplishing your goals. Whether you are watching your streaks grow, building new recipes, writing out your weekly menu and/

or recording your workouts, the templates and worksheets found in the additional health and wellness asset supplements will help you increase fitness value and take you to the next level. The New Habits Streak and Your Measurements logs are included in this journal. If you are interested in receiving additional assets please visit **infamousmothers.com** for more information.

Finally, use Covet to connect the dots between your data, day-to-day experiences and other parts of your wellness walk. Numbers, like your weight, are important. Numbers read within the context of your life are powerful and can encourage major transformations.

Remember, you are powerful alone but more impactful within a community. For this reason, we have created weekly workshops, quarterly retreats and other spaces to bring you in contact with a community who will walk alongside you, encourage you and lovingly hold you accountable as you build out this new lifestyle, accomplish your milestones and fulfill your biggest health and wellness goals.

About Each Section

Gratitude

The daily gratitude prompts you will encounter are not run-of-the mill. They are meant to be sassy, bold, funny, and challenging as much as they are both aspirational and inspirational. Each day, you are invited to fill in the blanks to create a statement of gratitude about some aspect of your life.

Dirty Word

Each gratitude prompt at the top of the page is paired with a "dirty word" quote at the bottom. I call it this, in part, because sometimes we are appropriating inspiration that was never meant for us and sometimes we are drawing inspiration from sources that mainstream would not accept as appropriate.

Quiet as Kept

On the third day of every week, look forward to a personal (and sometimes vulnerable) tip shared with you by either a fellow member, one of our instructors or a friend of the Covet program. You will find them on the bottom of the Daily Shit page. Whereas dirty words are often quotes from famous people or published works, tips offered in this section are from people who are directly connected to the health and wellness industry and/or specifically connected to the Covet program.

Goals

We can't stress this enough: Goals written down are more likely to be accomplished than goals that never leave our brains. With this in mind, Covet offers you several opportunities to commit to your goals, to repeat and tweak those goals—IN WRITING.

Our intention is to keep those important milestones in front of you. It is to remind you to celebrate your achievements, learn from any setbacks and keep you focused when distractions and life want to pull you in directions that do not serve your purposes. Having these final results in mind encourages us to build new behaviors and can give us what we need to sustain momentum. It can also give us a sense of accomplishment.

As you establish your goals, we recommend that you use the S.M.A.R.T.E.R. system. S.M.A.R.T.E.R. is an acronym for specific, measurable, achievable, relevant, timely, evaluate, and re-adjust. We will explore this more in our retreat.

Finally, as you begin planning your goals, remember that they should consider all aspects of your being: physical, emotional, spiritual and mental. You do not have to establish a goal for each, however, we do recommend that you explore your whole person as you begin thinking about how you want to move forward.

Weekly Goals

Weekly goals are the building blocks and smaller components of 4-week goals. Each week is meant to move you strategically to your 4-week milestone. You can focus on one thing, or you can work on building a new micro-habit each week. Your strategy will depend on your needs and your larger goals.

Daily Goals

Daily goals are the building blocks of weekly ones, and they are the most critical to your success. If big-picture goals are the foundation on which all others are created, the daily ones are the foundation on which all others will be accomplished. The success of your future aims rest on your ability to be strategic about today, to be flexible and resilient, and to learn and recover from any setbacks on a day-to-day basis. Your success depends on your ability to recognize that your plans for the future have been laid down so thoughtfully and strategically by you that you can focus on the right now, knowing that you can adjust as you see fit.

Daily Shit

The journey to a healthier, more fit version of yourselves can feel like anything but "polite" and "proper." It can be messy, chaotic, unpredictable, and frustrating. It can feel empowering, overwhelming, inspiring, and discouraging—a roller coaster of highs and lows that swings us from moments of deep pride to moments of extreme doubt. And while we know the long-term benefits of trusting the process, staying the course and sticking with the plan right now may mean you need to drop a few four-letter words.

While profanity has historically been seen as unrefined and immoral behavior, research shows that there might be some benefits, including ones associated with health, that come with cussing. Swearing has been associated with better workout performances, "increased circulation, elevated endorphins, and an overall sense of calm, control, and well-being."[1] Science also reveals that people who swear might be more honest. This is particularly important as so much of our success on this health and wellness journey depends on our ability to reflect genuinely and hold ourselves and our peers accountable.

With science on your side, use the section "I'm the Shit" to brag shamelessly about what you are "winning at" each day. Record your successes, moments of vanity, new discoveries, etc. This is where you declare yourself awesome, where you bust through your box and choose not to be small so that other people can be comfortable. This is where you defy convention by refusing to be "humble." Instead of waiting another second—or worse, a lifetime—to receive validation from someone else, by stating that you are the shit and reminding yourself of all the reasons why this is true, you will build a daily ritual of validating yourself. This is particularly important and empowering for women and people of color who remind ourselves daily that our "shine is not for the shade." We close out this section by sharing how we plan to build on our successes or reward ourselves just for living and breathing badassery.

Use the section "This Is Some Bullshit" to vent and face head-on the challenges that come your way on this journey. Write honestly about obstacles and barriers you encounter, fears, failures, disappointments, and frustrations. Record moments when you feel uninspired. This is the place you can openly, without apology, guilt, or shame, own your "ugly feelings," your unflattering thoughts and insecurities. And after you put it all out there, it's the place you strategize about how to move forward, how to use these experiences as fuel that can sustain you along the way, because nothing is wasted—EVER.

Monthly Shit

At the end of each 4-week session, you will have an opportunity to check in on your self-confidence and self-value. These two check points make up the section of the journal called Monthly Shit.

1 https://www.huffpost.com/entry/health-benefits-of-swearing_n_5a5e44a8e4b0106b7f65b3a6

Self-Value Tank

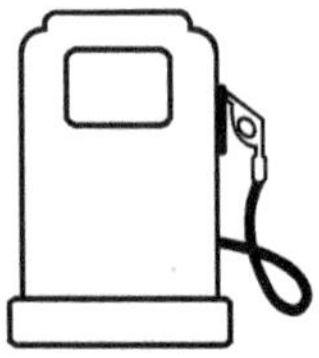

When I was younger, I remember hearing women saying to each other (and sometimes to me), "Girl, you gotta love yourself." They'd say it to a woman who was trying to recover from the devastation of a broken heart. "Girl, don't worry about his sorry ass. You gotta love you." They would say it to a woman who was what they'd call promiscuous. "Uh uh, you out here sleeping with this one and that one. That's because you don't love YOU." They'd say it to a woman struggling after having too many kids. "When are you going to start loving you?" For some reason, hearing that always felt more like an indictment or as if the receiver of this advice was being looked down upon more than it felt encouraging. Over time, I learned to hate hearing women say that to each other because no one ever explained what it meant or showed me and the people to whom that advice was directed what "loving ourselves" looked like. But as I grew, I also learned that part of the problem was that love was always understood as a noun, an emotion. When it was introduced to me as a verb, an action word, it began to "hit" differently. That was some years ago.

Today, I find myself learning a similar lesson with the word *self-value*. Often, we understand it as a thing, a feeling. But it is more than how we feel about ourselves. "Self-value is 'more behavioral than emotional, more about how you act toward what you value, including yourself, than how you feel about yourself compared to others.'"[2] Like *love, value* is both a noun and a verb. Self-value is displayed in how we handle ourselves, the appreciation we show ourselves, and the care we extend to ourselves. Together, all of these actions speak to the value we've placed on our bodies, minds, spirits, and hearts. To be clear, I am not an expert on these terms. I'm not a psychologist. I am, however, fascinated by the idea of self-value being more about how we behave than how we feel. As you progress through your health and wellness journey, at the end of each 4-week session, you will be invited to look back over the work you've done and reflect on what actions you have taken toward honoring your wellness walk. Your answers may include anything from committing to regular workouts, protecting your "me time," protecting your sleep, etc. Each month, hopefully, you will be able to identify for yourself how you've either maintained self-value or grown in it.

As you embark on this journey to trim your waists, fall in love with yourselves again, and grow stronger, your goal is to also grow in self-value. It is to develop behaviors that suggest your health and wellness deserve respect, protection, and investment. You will use this section of the journal as a tool to help you not only stay mindful about building and maintaining strong practices around your goals in these areas, it will also help you identify areas where you may believe you're prioritizing your wellness, but your actions are suggesting something else. I cannot stress this important factor enough: the purpose of this exercise is to offer you a tool that allows you to connect the dots and reflect on the link between what you say you value and what your actions are demonstrating. It is not meant to be used to determine your self-worth or even judge yourself—either favorably or unfavorably.

2 https://positivepsychology.com/self-worth/

Self-Confidence Scale

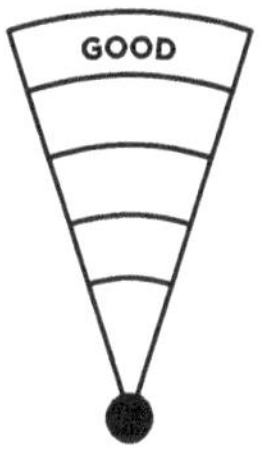

The dictionary defines self-confidence as "a feeling of trust in one's abilities, qualities, and judgment." Within the context of your work here, the focus is on these two key words: feeling and trust. Do you feel that you can trust yourself to meet your health and wellness goals? Do you believe you have what it takes to build healthy habits and to transform your life in a way that allows you to become the best version of yourself? More importantly, in the areas that challenge you most, do you trust yourself to learn to overcome and build (or maintain) the discipline to overcome those challenges? Confidence is going to be crucial to your success. Each month, you will be invited to check in with your self-confidence using a rating scale. You will then have the option to briefly reflect on your assessment in writing as part of Monthly Shit.

Weekly Goals

Minding My Weekly Business

At the start of every week is a section of your journal called "Minding My Weekly Business." Here you are invited to think about and predict the character of your upcoming week. Will you be busier than usual? Is your cycle coming on? Is it a routine week? Once you have identified two major features of your upcoming week, you are asked to focus on a strategy. These include, for example, meal prep, spicing up your routine, avoiding self-sabotage, managing triggers, etc. This section is particularly important because it asks you to identify your support for the week. Based on what you understand about the week ahead of you, who do you believe are the folks, groups, etc., that can help you be successful? This last part of Minding My Weekly Business is particularly important. Oftentimes, we include in our support network people we want to support us versus people who can either be supportive or are supportive. There is a difference. That difference plays out in your success.

The Weekly Preview

Each new week begins with an invitation for you to map out the upcoming seven days. This section of your journal is called "The Weekly Preview." It is designed to help you create a snapshot of what you hope to accomplish that week with regard to your physical activity, spirituality, emotions, mental health, self-care, and food goals.

Each Weekly Preview begins with a check-in meant to bring awareness to where you stand with regard to self-esteem. Not to be confused with self-confidence, although the two terms are often used interchangeably, self-esteem is understood as "a person's overall subjective sense of personal worth or value."[3] Self-esteem is important because it can influence your decision making and motivate you to take on new challenges.[4] For people who identify as women and people of color, it is particularly important that you check in with your perceptions of your value and worth as the racism, discrimination, and microaggressions that you may face daily can have a negative impact, shaping the choices you make on your health and wellness journey. Awareness of where you stand regarding your

3 "What is Self-Esteem?" Kendra Cherry, Verywellmind, April 24, 2021.

4 See above

self-esteem can help you challenge yourself during weeks you are considering playing small and inspire you to keep owning your boss status on weeks you are "feeling yourself." Healthy self-esteem will help you reach your health and wellness goals because it allows you to accept that you deserve to be well in every way.

Weeklies: The Building Blocks of 4-Week Goals

While weekly goals are the building blocks of 4-week goals, they are also where you start to become more detailed and focused. As you begin to establish your weekly goals, ask yourself these questions, "What are all the things I need to do to successfully reach my 4-week plan? What new habits do I need to build? What behaviors do I need to change? What larger systemic issues are operating in my life, and how are they impacting me? How can I turn things to my advantage, even when I seem to be at a disadvantage?" With the information you currently have, create an exhaustive list. One way to do this is by creating a "habit web." This is inspired by the "word web" often used in classrooms to help students gain an understanding of vocabulary by comparing, contrasting, and building other associations in the form of a web.

With this in mind, put your "primary habits" or the major habits you are looking to develop (see 4-week goals) at the center of your web. Start creating a list of behaviors and activities associated with these. Do this until you feel you have a clear sense of what behaviors and habits you will need to establish and build to make it possible for you to reach the goals at the center of the web. To get a better idea, see the following example:

HABIT WEB

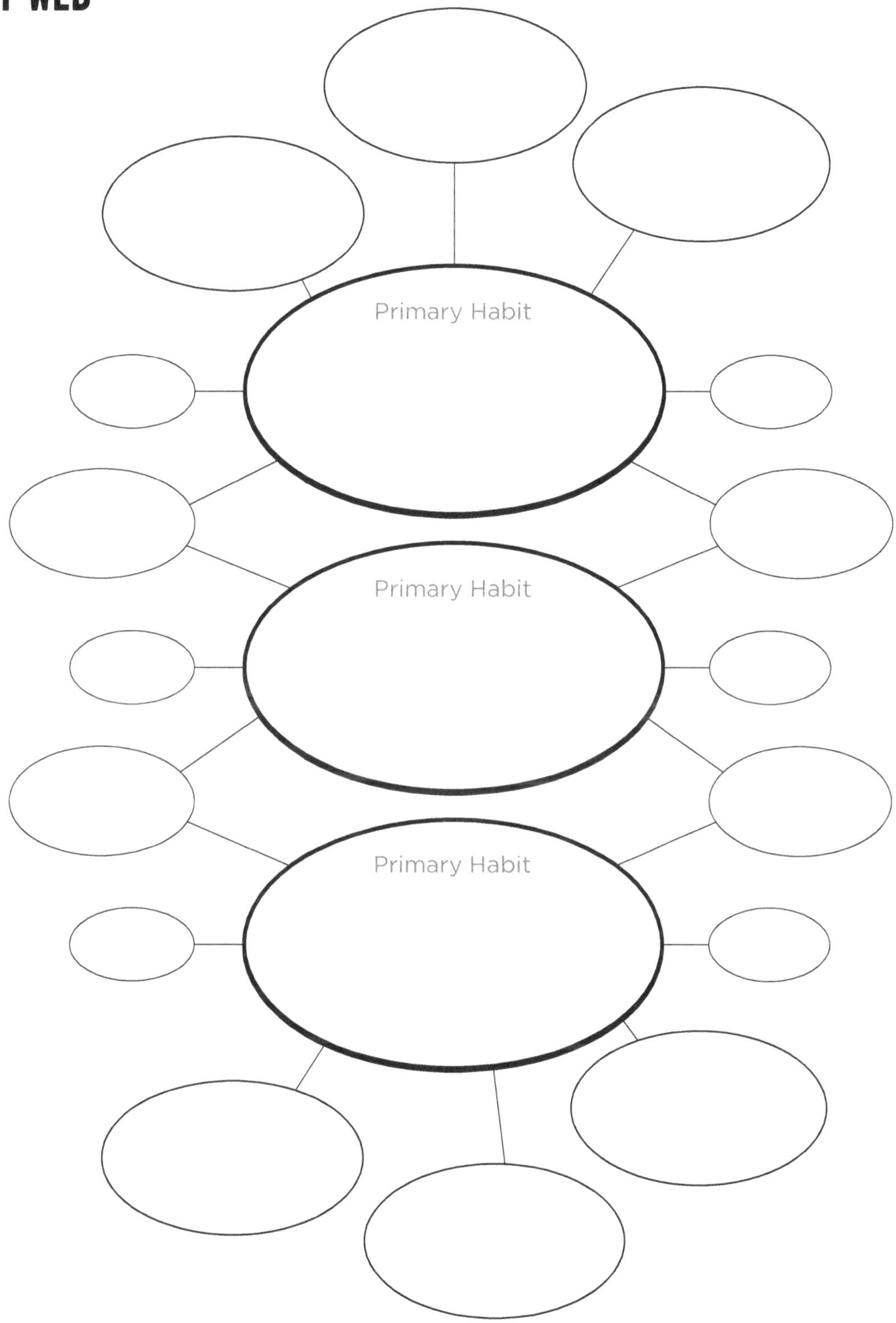

Once your Habit Web is complete, refine the goals by listing them in the chart below.

Goal 1:

How will I accomplish Goal 1:

Goal 2:

How will I accomplish Goal 2:

Goal 3:

How will I accomplish Goal 3:

Once you've completed this exercise, identify the behaviors you believe you can begin making significant progress on within a week. Example: A woman, we'll call her Shantel, wants to be in bed by 9:00 p.m. each weeknight. To accomplish this, the following actions will need to become habits:

- She needs to make sure dinner is prepared and completed between 6:30 and 7:00 p.m.
- She needs to have a wind-down routine that encourages her children and/or herself to calm down before bed and have a restful night.
- Shantel needs to have her children in bed and asleep by 8:30 p.m.

Whew! This is a lot and totally doable with the right mindset, community, and strategies in place. Currently, her children go to bed at 11:00 p.m. So her strategy might be to start putting them to bed 30 minutes earlier each night until she reaches 8:00 or 8:15, with the goal of them being asleep by 8:30. Or, her strategy might be to wake up her children at 5:00 a.m. every morning, 2.5 hours earlier than normal, so that they get tired sooner. As part of the wind-down part of her children's new sleep schedule, she realizes that electronics should be off in her home. So she has decided to do something very simple and radical at the same time: CUT OFF WiFi by 7:00 p.m.! She also has to find a way to fill what was once their screen time with something relaxing that will lead to a restful night's sleep. Her action plan for the week could look something like this:

- Wake children up by 5:00 a.m.
- Cut off WiFi seven nights a week by 7:00 p.m.
- Bathe children between 7:15 p.m. and 7:45 p.m. (Sunday through Thursday)
- Children read their favorite story from 7:50 p.m. to 8:00 p.m. (Sunday through Thursday)
- At 8:00 p.m., play relaxing music (Sunday through Saturday)

Week after week, Shantel focuses on mastering this plan until it's time to graduate to a new one. As the weeks go by, and as her family gets comfortable with this new schedule, she can begin to make adjustments as she sees fit. For example, once they conquer this schedule, she may want to add an evening walk before dinner. Prior to calling the kids in for the night, the family may take a lap around the block to help everyone switch gears from outside time to inside time.

While the focus has been on getting the children asleep by 8:30, this week's goal has been in service of Shantel's own goal of being in bed by 9:00 p.m. within the next four weeks. In addition, many of the strategies in place for her children can also be applied to her routine. These include turning off WiFi, waking up earlier, and playing relaxing music. By centering their needs, she is not delaying her own. On the contrary, she directly benefits from the schedule she is building for her family AND doing the work it takes to get closer to her primary goals.

Another thing to consider as you set your goals is your schedule, events, and overall week's character. This week, are you traveling more or less, going on vacation, busier than usual, less busy, recovering, getting back to your routine, injured, feeding additional mouths, feeding mouths? Be mindful of your week's character, and plan with that in mind, as much as you consider your goals. This will help set yourself up for success and help you identify opportunities offered in some weeks that are not present in others (and vice versa).

Finally, be mindful of what you are focusing on this week: water intake, activity, sleep, meal planning, tracking, staying within calorie/point count, steps, mindfulness, etc. Commit to up to three focal points.

Daily Goals

If you've guessed that daily goals are the building blocks of weekly goals, you've been paying attention to the pattern, and you are 100 percent correct. The goals you establish day-to-day are meant to help you accomplish your weekly milestones. This means that you will look to those milestones to understand what you should be aiming for each day. Instead of "winging it," your hours have more specific assignments, tasks that now serve the higher purpose of helping you reach your health and wellness goals. This means your activities will fall into one of three categories: building on what's working, organic changes, utilitarian changes and micro-habits.

Build on What's Working

On a day-to-day basis, you are already winning on so many levels. It's time to take your boss-woman ways to new heights. Let's say you have been working around the clock to care for the kids and increase your company's bottom line. You walk past the mirror, and the struggle shows in your appearance. You've been taking care of everyone and everything for so long, you don't even know where to start reclaiming your sass and shine. But actually, you do. Start with what's working. It can't be all bad—even when we think it is. So capture that part of yourself that is peeking out her resilient face and start there. It could be your refusal to let go of your manicures. Okay, now add some rings to those fingers. It could be those beautiful lips that stand out no matter what. Well, gloss them up, girl! It could be your commitment to sitting in the car in the parking lot for some alone time. Now use that time to create a mood board on your phone through Pinterest, for example, designing your new look. And then follow through with it. Unlike "organic changes," building on what's working is not always a natural next step—even though it can be in this context. It is using what you are already doing successfully as a springboard for more success.

Organic Changes

Like the build-on-what's-working technique, organic changes are all about finding activities that you have either mastered or established a strong routine for and using that as a building block to up the ante. But unlike the former technique, this one is an obvious progression on what you are already doing.

One way to make an organic change is to look for ways to repeat exactly what you are currently doing. For example, you already work out two days a week, on Monday and Wednesday at 6:00 a.m., and you love it! So adding a Friday workout may be a "natural next step." You have the space available in your schedule, you have already built the discipline of working out, and you know it's going to give you the results you crave regarding strength, weight loss, and energy.

Another way you can make an organic change is by taking things to the natural next level. You've been taking a beginner's flow yoga class for over a year. You're comfortable with it and have a solid foundation. Start taking the intermediate one. It takes place on Tuesday and Thursday every week, from 12:00 to 1:00 p.m., and it fulfills your weekly goal of practicing. It's a logical next step. After all, you set a long-term goal of becoming an advanced yogi within three years.

Utilitarian Change

Another change we're considering here will be referred to as "utilitarian change." Unlike organic changes, this action is often not natural for us. Utilitarian, by definition, means something is designed to be useful or practical over attractive. To make choices that are useful and practical over the ones that "look" good is not always an innate move for many of us. And yet, our goal is for it to become second nature to choose the option that gets us to the milestones we have prioritized in our weekly action plan when presented with competing and overwhelming possibilities. If the tasks you have to choose between are both in service of items in your action plan, choose an option that either serves both, if that's possible, or choose the option that gets you to the milestone that has the greatest impact on your progress.

Consider this scenario. You've decided that every day you'll run three miles. But you missed your morning run because you had to start your workday earlier than usual. To fulfill your task, you plan to run before dinner. You then realize that doing so might get in the way of your night schedule, which can then get in the way of your goal of being in bed by 8:30 p.m. so you can get up by 4:30 a.m. to write and then run. You have to make some choices. Do you shorten your run to less than your usual one hour so that you can stick to your routine? Do you forgo the run? Whatever choice you make, it must be in service of your bigger goal of getting a good night's sleep. You choose the second option because you know that running for 45 minutes won't sit well with you. You need the whole hour. Not to mention, you will need a cool-off period of about 15 minutes, and you will need to shower. The more you think about this, you see this run jeopardizing the milestone that matters most to you, which is your sleep and wake-up schedule. To honor your cardio goal, you've decided to use this day as one of your two days off this week.

Sometimes utilitarian choices can feel like a sacrifice. A slight perspective shift can help de-emphasize the idea of surrendering something in place of something else. Instead, emphasize the reality of you being a badass who makes boss decisions that honor where you are going. For example, consider a woman named Arya. For Arya to accomplish her goals, she needs six more hours in her schedule each week. With her current life the way it is, it's impossible to squeeze blood from this turnip. As she racks her brain, it dawns on her that it takes her exactly six hours to twist her hair every week. Right then and there, she decides to grab the hair clippers, and she shaves off her thick coils. After all, she has been thinking about cutting her hair for some time now. This seems like the perfect opportunity to do so. She has instantly created six hours in her schedule, allowing her to fulfill her weekly goal of meditation three times a week and meal prep.

Micro Habits

We can't talk about daily goals without dedicating space to behaviors called micro-habits. A micro-habit is an action that requires little motivation and effort to complete. Regularly doing this small activity leads to longer commitments that turn into full-blown habits over time. How can you tell the difference between a micro-habit and an actual habit? Micro-habits are the baby steps (usually starting with one step) that lead to the development of the big habit. Also, micro-habits should be completed in under one to two minutes.

They should be connected with something you care about, and the effort to do them should be so small you cannot fail. If your goal is to drink half of your weight in ounces of water every day for 21 days, but you hate drinking water, you can start with the micro-habit of drinking one sip of water with dinner for seven days straight. If your goal is to brush your teeth every night, commit to brushing your tongue after dinner. Or, if you want to commit to walking 10,000 steps a day, jump on the treadmill and walk 100 steps after you shower in the morning. In each of these examples, you are committing to an act so small that it takes very little effort on your part, you are connecting the activity with a routine you do daily, and you can accomplish it in under one to two minutes.

With this in mind, let's revisit Shantel's example for the final time. Although she knows dinner is an important part of her children's ability to successfully stick to their night-time schedule, she struggles to see how she can prepare dinner early. She loves to cook for her family, but she doesn't have the time since launching her new startup. In this new schedule she is creating, she has slotted dinner (including cooking and eating) from 6:30 p.m. to 7:15 p.m. because it makes sense with the flow of her schedule. She doesn't know how she is going to accomplish this. Enter the micro-habit.

Instead of cooking an elaborate meal, Shantel can commit to meals that take under two minutes of effort, such as salads, sandwiches, pizza, etc. Remember, the goal is to prepare a meal for her and her children, which makes it effortless for her to build the habit of having dinner on the table and completed within the time frame she has allotted. Once she has established this habit, she can plan for more complex meals or meals that will require more advanced preparation, if she chooses.

Today's goals...

Habit	Goals	Outcomes
Sleep		
Water		
Food		
Fitness		
Steps		
Stress		
Habit: ____________		
Habit: ____________		
Habit: ____________		

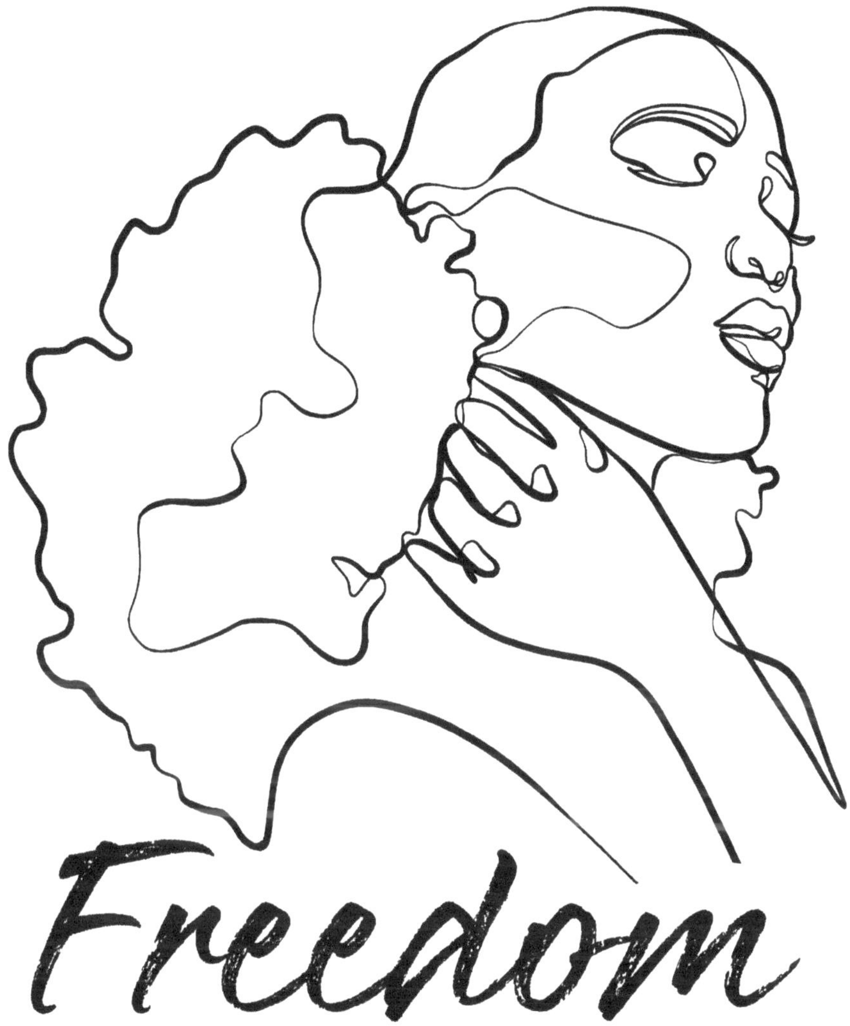

Freedom

"It is our duty to fight for our freedom. It is our duty to win.
We must love each other and support each other.
We have nothing to lose but our chains."

-Assata Shakur

Weeks 1-4

Week 1

Minding My Weekly Business

Crystal ball, what does my upcoming week look like? (choose up to two):

- ❍ In these streets, on these interstates—everywhere but home
- ❍ Recommitting to my health and wellness goals—getting back on plan
- ❍ You know the routine
- ❍ A schedule that is super crazy
- ❍ Me time that doesn't include working on my plan
- ❍ Approaching goal or milestone
- ❍ My cycle is coming/I'm on my cycle
- ❍ I am living with the symptoms of perimenopause/menopause.
- ❍ ______________________________

Now that I have stared into my future, I will commit to focusing on the following (choose up to two):

- ❍ Meal and snack prep
- ❍ A mindset that leads me to success
- ❍ Spice up my routine
- ❍ Stay calm, stay focused, stay relaxed
- ❍ Mindful eating in these streets, on these interstates
- ❍ Meet my sleep goals
- ❍ Move my body more
- ❍ Eat within calorie/points budget
- ❍ Avoid self-sabotage
- ❍ Manage triggers
- ❍ Stay in community, attend meetings, get coaching
- ❍ Manage the symptoms associated with my cycle
- ❍ Meet myself where I am in this new season of life
- ❍ ______________________________

This week, my support includes:

____

____

Weekly Preview

Rosenberg Self-Esteem Scale (Rosenberg-SES)

Below is a list of statements dealing with your general feelings about yourself.

Complete these questions based upon your feelings.

1.	On the whole, I am satisfied with myself.
2.	*At times, I think I am no good at all.
3.	I feel that I have a number of good qualities.
4.	I am able to do things as well as most other people.
5.	*I feel I do not have much to be proud of.
6.	*I certainly feel useless at times.
7.	I feel that I'm a person of worth, at least on an equal plane with others.
8.	*I wish I could have more respect for myself.
9.	*All in all, I am inclined to feel that I am a failure.
10.	I take a positive attitude toward myself.

Scoring

Strongly agree = 3;

Agree = 2;

Disagree = 1;

Strongly disagree = 0.

*Items with an asterisk are reverse scored. To calculate the total self-esteem score, sum the scores for the 10 items. The higher the score, the higher the self-esteem.

Score	Level of Self Esteem
0-10	Low
11-20	Moderate
21-30	High

©The Morris Rosenberg Foundation; c/o Department of Sociology; University of Maryland; 2112 Art/Soc Building; College Park, MD 20742-1315

	Strongly Disagree	Disagree	Agree	Strongly Agree

Weekly Goals

This graph is designed to help you create a snapshot of what you hope to accomplish that week.

Focus	**Sun.**	**Mon.**	**Tues.**	
Physical				
Mental				
Emotional				
Spiritual				
Self Care				
Breakfast				
Lunch				
Dinner				
Snacks				

	Wed.	Thurs.	Fri.	Sat.

Day 1
Week 1

A DIRTY WORD

"What's the world for you if you can't make it up the way you want it?"

-Toni Morrison, author of *Jazz*

Today's goals...

Habit	Goals	Outcomes
Sleep		
Water		
Food		
Fitness		
Steps		
Stress		
Habit: ____________		
Habit: ____________		
Habit: ____________		

A MOMENT OF GRATITUDE

I am grateful that I have the power to make up my world the way I want it. So far, I have used my power to (re)create my space in this way

Daily Shit: Reflections about Today's Goals and Outcomes

I'm the **SHIT** because:

I am proud of this because:

This is how I am going to build on that:

Today's **BULLSHIT** is this:

I feel frustrated, disappointed, angry, discouraged

[insert appropriate feeling here]

because:

Here is my solution to this bullshit:

Day 2
Week 1

A DIRTY WORD

"We're all capable of climbing so much higher than we usually permit ourselves to suppose."

-Octavia Butler, author of *Blood Child*

Today's goals...

Habit	Goals	Outcomes
Sleep		
Water		
Food		
Fitness		
Steps		
Stress		
Habit: ____________		
Habit: ____________		
Habit: ____________		

A MOMENT OF GRATITUDE

I am grateful that I have climbed higher than I usually permit myself in the following area(s) of my life

____

[insert the area in which you have climbed higher].

Daily Shit: Reflections about Today's Goals and Outcomes

I'm the **SHIT** because:

I am proud of this because:

This is how I am going to build on that:

Today's **BULLSHIT** is this:

I feel frustrated, disappointed, angry, discouraged

[insert appropriate feeling here]

because:

Here is my solution to this bullshit:

Day 3
Week 1

A DIRTY WORD

"Better to stay alive," I said. "At least while there's a chance to get free."

~Octavia Butler, author of *Kindred*

Today's goals...

Habit	Goals	Outcomes
Sleep		
Water		
Food		
Fitness		
Steps		
Stress		
Habit: ____________		
Habit: ____________		
Habit: ____________		

A MOMENT OF GRATITUDE

I am grateful that I stayed alive when a thousand things tried to kill me. One thing I have overcome is

____

[insert your answer above]

QUIET AS KEPT

"Make a change today that you will thank yourself for a year from now."

~Precious "Coach P" Woodley, Me2You Selfcare Enterprise, Madison, WI

Daily Shit: Reflections about Today's Goals and Outcomes

I'm the **SHIT** because:

I am proud of this because:

This is how I am going to build on that:

Today's **BULLSHIT** is this:

I feel frustrated, disappointed, angry, discouraged

[insert appropriate feeling here]

because:

Here is my solution to this bullshit:

Day 4
Week 1

A DIRTY WORD

"I shall create! If not a note, a hole. If not an overture, a desecration."
~Gwendolyn Brooks

Today's goals...

Habit	Goals	Outcomes
Sleep		
Water		
Food		
Fitness		
Steps		
Stress		
Habit: ____________		
Habit: ____________		
Habit: ____________		

A MOMENT OF GRATITUDE

I shall create! If not something constructive, like a

[insert something you can build], then I will destroy

[insert something you can tear down]. I am grateful that I am aware of my power to both build or destroy.

Daily Shit: Reflections about Today's Goals and Outcomes

I'm the **SHIT** because:

I am proud of this because:

This is how I am going to build on that:

Today's **BULLSHIT** is this:

I feel frustrated, disappointed, angry, discouraged

[insert appropriate feeling here]

because:

Here is my solution to this bullshit:

Day 5
Week 1

A DIRTY WORD

"When I dare to be powerful, to use my strength in the service of my vision, then it becomes less and less important whether I am afraid."

-Audre Lorde

Today's goals...

Habit	Goals	Outcomes
Sleep		
Water		
Food		
Fitness		
Steps		
Stress		
Habit: ____________		
Habit: ____________		
Habit: ____________		

A MOMENT OF GRATITUDE

I am grateful that I dared to be powerful, to use my strength in service of my vision to

____

[insert your vision] and it doesn't matter that I was afraid.

Daily Shit: Reflections about Today's Goals and Outcomes

I'm the **SHIT** because:

I am proud of this because:

This is how I am going to build on that:

Today's **BULLSHIT** is this:

I feel frustrated, disappointed, angry, discouraged

[insert appropriate feeling here]

because:

Here is my solution to this bullshit:

Day 6
Week 1

A DIRTY WORD

"Can't nothing make your life work if you ain't the architect."
~Terry McMillan

Today's goals...

Habit	Goals	Outcomes
Sleep		
Water		
Food		
Fitness		
Steps		
Stress		
Habit: ____________		
Habit: ____________		
Habit: ____________		

A MOMENT OF GRATITUDE

I am grateful that I have the freedom to design my life. I have used that freedom to (re)create the life I want by

____

[insert your answer].

Daily Shit: Reflections about Today's Goals and Outcomes

I'm the **SHIT** because:

I am proud of this because:

This is how I am going to build on that:

Today's **BULLSHIT** is this:

I feel frustrated, disappointed, angry, discouraged

[insert appropriate feeling here]

because:

Here is my solution to this bullshit:

Day 7
Week 1

A DIRTY WORD

"You're not going to succeed unless you believe that your way of doing things is as right as anybody else's."

-Nathalie Molina Niño

Today's goals...

Habit	Goals	Outcomes
Sleep		
Water		
Food		
Fitness		
Steps		
Stress		
Habit: ___________		
Habit: ___________		
Habit: ___________		

A MOMENT OF GRATITUDE

I know that my way of

____

[insert something you are working on, a problem you are solving, etc].is just as good as, if not better than, anybody else's way. I am grateful for the freedom to innovate.

Daily Shit: Reflections about Today's Goals and Outcomes

I'm the **SHIT** because:

I am proud of this because:

This is how I am going to build on that:

Today's **BULLSHIT** is this:

I feel frustrated, disappointed, angry, discouraged

[insert appropriate feeling here]

because:

Here is my solution to this bullshit:

THE WEEKLY TEA ... SPILL IT

What are you most proud of this week?

What challenged you this week?

What lessons will you take with you into next week?

Week 2

Minding My Weekly Business

Crystal ball, what does my upcoming week look like? (choose up to two):

- ❍ In these streets, on these interstates—everywhere but home
- ❍ Recommitting to my health and wellness goals—getting back on plan
- ❍ You know the routine
- ❍ A schedule that is super crazy
- ❍ Me time that doesn't include working on my plan
- ❍ Approaching goal or milestone
- ❍ My cycle is coming/I'm on my cycle
- ❍ I am living with the symptoms of perimenopause/menopause.
- ❍ ______________________________

Now that I have stared into my future, I will commit to focusing on the following (choose up to two):

- ❍ Meal and snack prep
- ❍ A mindset that leads me to success
- ❍ Spice up my routine
- ❍ Stay calm, stay focused, stay relaxed
- ❍ Mindful eating in these streets, on these interstates
- ❍ Meet my sleep goals
- ❍ Move my body more
- ❍ Eat within calorie/points budget
- ❍ Avoid self-sabotage
- ❍ Manage triggers
- ❍ Stay in community, attend meetings, get coaching
- ❍ Manage the symptoms associated with my cycle
- ❍ Meet myself where I am in this new season of life
- ❍ ______________________________

This week, my support includes:

____

____

Weekly Preview

Rosenberg Self-Esteem Scale (Rosenberg-SES)

Below is a list of statements dealing with your general feelings about yourself.

Complete these questions based upon your feelings.

1.	On the whole, I am satisfied with myself.
2.	*At times, I think I am no good at all.
3.	I feel that I have a number of good qualities.
4.	I am able to do things as well as most other people.
5.	*I feel I do not have much to be proud of.
6.	*I certainly feel useless at times.
7.	I feel that I'm a person of worth, at least on an equal plane with others.
8.	*I wish I could have more respect for myself.
9.	*All in all, I am inclined to feel that I am a failure.
10.	I take a positive attitude toward myself.

Scoring

Strongly agree = 3;

Agree = 2;

Disagree = 1;

Strongly disagree = 0.

*Items with an asterisk are reverse scored. To calculate the total self-esteem score, sum the scores for the 10 items. The higher the score, the higher the self-esteem.

Score	Level of Self Esteem
0-10	Low
11-20	Moderate
21-30	High

©The Morris Rosenberg Foundation; c/o Department of Sociology; University of Maryland; 2112 Art/Soc Building; College Park, MD 20742-1315

	Strongly Disagree	Disagree	Agree	Strongly Agree

Weekly Goals

This graph is designed to help you create a snapshot of what you hope to accomplish that week.

Focus	Sun.	Mon.	Tues.
Physical			
Mental			
Emotional			
Spiritual			
Self Care			
Breakfast			
Lunch			
Dinner			
Snacks			

Wed.	Thurs.	Fri.	Sat.

Day 1
Week 2

A DIRTY WORD

"I pay attention. I ask myself what it is about this person I am coveting. How can I acquire it? How can I learn from it?"

-Nely Galán

Today's goals...

Habit	Goals	Outcomes
Sleep		
Water		
Food		
Fitness		
Steps		
Stress		
Habit: ______________		
Habit: ______________		
Habit: ______________		

A MOMENT OF GRATITUDE

I covet these three qualities:

1. ______________________________

2. ______________________________

3. ______________________________

from my future self. I am grateful for the woman I will become.

Daily Shit: Reflections about Today's Goals and Outcomes

I'm the **SHIT** because:

I am proud of this because:

This is how I am going to build on that:

Today's **BULLSHIT** is this:

I feel frustrated, disappointed, angry, discouraged

[insert appropriate feeling here]

because:

Here is my solution to this bullshit:

Day 2
Week 2

A DIRTY WORD

"Nothing is impossible; the word itself says 'I'm possible'!"

~Audrey Hepburn

Today's goals...

Habit	Goals	Outcomes
Sleep		
Water		
Food		
Fitness		
Steps		
Stress		
Habit: ____________		
Habit: ____________		
Habit: ____________		

A MOMENT OF GRATITUDE

I thought it was impossible to

____

[insert accomplishment]. I am grateful that I believed in myself enough to do something that was once my wildest dream.

Daily Shit: Reflections about Today's Goals and Outcomes

I'm the **SHIT** because:

I am proud of this because:

This is how I am going to build on that:

Today's **BULLSHIT** is this:

I feel frustrated, disappointed, angry, discouraged

[insert appropriate feeling here]

because:

Here is my solution to this bullshit:

Day 3
Week 2

A DIRTY WORD

"I wrote the book in order to give myself permission." -Terry McMillan

Today's goals...

Habit	Goals	Outcomes
Sleep		
Water		
Food		
Fitness		
Steps		
Stress		
Habit: ____________		
Habit: ____________		
Habit: ____________		

A MOMENT OF GRATITUDE

I am grateful for giving myself permission to

____

[insert what you've given yourself to permission to either be or do].

I feel more empowered.

QUIET AS KEPT

"Get naked and stand in the mirror, looking at yourself completely naked and look yourself in the eyes, telling yourself, 'I love you

____

[insert your name]. I'm in love with you.' Do this every day until you know it to be true.

-Mistee Quinones, Tastee Gurlz, Chicago, IL

Daily Shit: Reflections about Today's Goals and Outcomes

I'm the **SHIT** because:

I am proud of this because:

This is how I am going to build on that:

Today's **BULLSHIT** is this:

I feel frustrated, disappointed, angry, discouraged

[insert appropriate feeling here]

because:

Here is my solution to this bullshit:

Day 4
Week 2

A DIRTY WORD

"You will wonder, 'Is this all there is? When will all of this work pay off? When do I get to have fun?' You will experience FOMO (fear of missing out). Don't get discouraged. I promise you the party is where you are because you are working and building something. Ask yourself, 'Do I want to spend the rest of my life watching what other people are doing? Or do I want to do what other people watch?' Think about that."

~Nely Galán

Today's goals...

Habit	Goals	Outcomes
Sleep		
Water		
Food		
Fitness		
Steps		
Stress		
Habit: ______		
Habit: ______		
Habit: ______		

A MOMENT OF GRATITUDE

I am grateful that I did not let the Fear of Missing Out (FOMO) conquer my life. I worked hard to

____

[insert accomplishment], and my life is better because I made that choice.

Daily Shit: Reflections about Today's Goals and Outcomes

I'm the **SHIT** because:

I am proud of this because:

This is how I am going to build on that:

Today's **BULLSHIT** is this:

I feel frustrated, disappointed, angry, discouraged

[insert appropriate feeling here]

because:

Here is my solution to this bullshit:

Day 5
Week 2

A DIRTY WORD

"The primary goal of the poor is survival, the aim of the middle class is *comfort,* and the objective of the wealthy is *freedom* and *control.*"

-Dennis Kimbro

Today's goals...

Habit	Goals	Outcomes
Sleep		
Water		
Food		
Fitness		
Steps		
Stress		
Habit: ____________		
Habit: ____________		
Habit: ____________		

A MOMENT OF GRATITUDE

I am grateful for my survival, for my comfort and, equally important, for my freedom. Freedom for me looks like this

____

[insert your vision of freedom].

Daily Shit: Reflections about Today's Goals and Outcomes

I'm the **SHIT** because:

I am proud of this because:

This is how I am going to build on that:

Today's **BULLSHIT** is this:

I feel frustrated, disappointed, angry, discouraged

[insert appropriate feeling here]

because:

Here is my solution to this bullshit:

Day 6
Week 2

A DIRTY WORD

"If you don't like the road you're walking, start paving another one."
~Dolly Parton

Today's goals...

Habit	Goals	Outcomes
Sleep		
Water		
Food		
Fitness		
Steps		
Stress		
Habit: ____________		
Habit: ____________		
Habit: ____________		

A MOMENT OF GRATITUDE

I didn't like the road I was on when I was

____

[insert a lifestyle choice or behavior], so I decided to change paths. And now I am

____

[insert the new event lifestyle choice or behavior].
I am grateful that I paved a new way.

Daily Shit: Reflections about Today's Goals and Outcomes

I'm the **SHIT** because:

I am proud of this because:

This is how I am going to build on that:

Today's **BULLSHIT** is this:

I feel frustrated, disappointed, angry, discouraged

[insert appropriate feeling here]

because:

Here is my solution to this bullshit:

Day 7
Week 2

A DIRTY WORD

"That it is still important to keep improving our lives, even at our age, and we should treat ourselves better and stop acting like our best years are behind us."

-Terry McMillan

Today's goals...

Habit	Goals	Outcomes
Sleep		
Water		
Food		
Fitness		
Steps		
Stress		
Habit: ____________		
Habit: ____________		
Habit: ____________		

A MOMENT OF GRATITUDE

I am grateful that I am still improving my life at the age of

____

[insert your age], because I know that the best years of my life are not behind me; they are right now.

Daily Shit: Reflections about Today's Goals and Outcomes

I'm the **SHIT** because:

I am proud of this because:

This is how I am going to build on that:

Today's **BULLSHIT** is this:

I feel frustrated, disappointed, angry, discouraged

[insert appropriate feeling here]

because:

Here is my solution to this bullshit:

THE WEEKLY TEA ... SPILL IT

What are you most proud of this week?

What challenged you this week?

What lessons will you take with you into next week?

Week 3

Minding My Weekly Business

Crystal ball, what does my upcoming week look like? (choose up to two):

- ❍ In these streets, on these interstates—everywhere but home
- ❍ Recommitting to my health and wellness goals—getting back on plan
- ❍ You know the routine
- ❍ A schedule that is super crazy
- ❍ Me time that doesn't include working on my plan
- ❍ Approaching goal or milestone
- ❍ My cycle is coming/I'm on my cycle
- ❍ I am living with the symptoms of perimenopause/menopause.
- ❍ ______________________________

Now that I have stared into my future, I will commit to focusing on the following (choose up to two):

- ❍ Meal and snack prep
- ❍ A mindset that leads me to success
- ❍ Spice up my routine
- ❍ Stay calm, stay focused, stay relaxed
- ❍ Mindful eating in these streets, on these interstates
- ❍ Meet my sleep goals
- ❍ Move my body more
- ❍ Eat within calorie/points budget
- ❍ Avoid self-sabotage
- ❍ Manage triggers
- ❍ Stay in community, attend meetings, get coaching
- ❍ Manage the symptoms associated with my cycle
- ❍ Meet myself where I am in this new season of life
- ❍ ______________________________

This week, my support includes:

____

____

Weekly Preview

Rosenberg Self-Esteem Scale (Rosenberg-SES)

Below is a list of statements dealing with your general feelings about yourself.
Complete these questions based upon your feelings.

1.	On the whole, I am satisfied with myself.
2.	*At times, I think I am no good at all.
3.	I feel that I have a number of good qualities.
4.	I am able to do things as well as most other people.
5.	*I feel I do not have much to be proud of.
6.	*I certainly feel useless at times.
7.	I feel that I'm a person of worth, at least on an equal plane with others.
8.	*I wish I could have more respect for myself.
9.	*All in all, I am inclined to feel that I am a failure.
10.	I take a positive attitude toward myself.

Scoring

Strongly agree = 3;
Agree = 2;
Disagree = 1;
Strongly disagree = 0.
*Items with an asterisk are reverse scored. To calculate the total self-esteem score, sum the scores for the 10 items. The higher the score, the higher the self-esteem.

Score	Level of Self Esteem
0-10	Low
11-20	Moderate
21-30	High

©The Morris Rosenberg Foundation; c/o Department of Sociology; University of Maryland; 2112 Art/Soc Building; College Park, MD 20742-1315

	Strongly Disagree	Disagree	Agree	Strongly Agree

Weekly Goals

This graph is designed to help you create a snapshot of what you hope to accomplish that week.

Focus	Sun.	Mon.	Tues.	
Physical				
Mental				
Emotional				
Spiritual				
Self Care				
Breakfast				
Lunch				
Dinner				
Snacks				

	Wed.	Thurs.	Fri.	Sat.

Day 1
Week 3

A DIRTY WORD

"Revolution is about change, and the first place the change begins is in yourself."
~Assata Shakur

Today's goals...

Habit	Goals	Outcomes
Sleep		
Water		
Food		
Fitness		
Steps		
Stress		
Habit: ____________		
Habit: ____________		
Habit: ____________		

A MOMENT OF GRATITUDE

I am grateful for the private revolution that is happening within me.
I have changed in these three ways:

1. ____________
2. ____________
3. ____________

Daily Shit: Reflections about Today's Goals and Outcomes

I'm the **SHIT** because:

I am proud of this because:

This is how I am going to build on that:

Today's **BULLSHIT** is this:

I feel frustrated, disappointed, angry, discouraged

[insert appropriate feeling here]

because:

Here is my solution to this bullshit:

Day 2
Week 3

A DIRTY WORD

"I think there are things for all of us to do as long as we're here and we're healthy."
~Gwendolyn Brooks

Today's goals...

Habit	Goals	Outcomes
Sleep		
Water		
Food		
Fitness		
Steps		
Stress		
Habit: ______		
Habit: ______		
Habit: ______		

A MOMENT OF GRATITUDE

I am grateful that I have the health to pursue these three things

1. ______
2. ______
3. ______

Daily Shit: Reflections about Today's Goals and Outcomes

I'm the **SHIT** because:

I am proud of this because:

This is how I am going to build on that:

Today's **BULLSHIT** is this:

I feel frustrated, disappointed, angry, discouraged

[insert appropriate feeling here]

because:

Here is my solution to this bullshit:

Day 3
Week 3

A DIRTY WORD

"Dreams are lovely but they are just dreams. Fleeting, ephemeral, pretty. But dreams do not come true just because you dream them. It's hard work that makes things happen. It's hard work that creates change." -Shonda Rhimes

Today's goals...

Habit	Goals	Outcomes
Sleep		
Water		
Food		
Fitness		
Steps		
Stress		
Habit: ____________		
Habit: ____________		
Habit: ____________		

A MOMENT OF GRATITUDE

I am grateful for my dream of

____

[insert your dream]. I am even more grateful for my ability to put in the work to make it happen.

QUIET AS KEPT

"At moments of mental health breakdown, if you can, find a reason to laugh. Watch a comedy, think of something funny—create an opportunity to laugh. It can be your best medicine."
-Tiffany Dews, Dews Group, Richmond

Daily Shit: Reflections about Today's Goals and Outcomes

I'm the **SHIT** because:

I am proud of this because:

This is how I am going to build on that:

Today's **BULLSHIT** is this:

I feel frustrated, disappointed, angry, discouraged

[insert appropriate feeling here]

because:

Here is my solution to this bullshit:

Day 4
Week 3

A DIRTY WORD

"I'm hungry for knowledge. The whole thing is to learn every day, to get brighter and brighter. That's what this world is about. You look at someone like Gandhi, and he glowed. Martin Luther King glowed. Muhammad Ali glows. I think that's from being bright all the time, and trying to be brighter."

~Jay-Z

Today's goals...

Habit	Goals	Outcomes
Sleep		
Water		
Food		
Fitness		
Steps		
Stress		
Habit: ______________		
Habit: ______________		
Habit: ______________		

A MOMENT OF GRATITUDE

I am brighter because I read

____

[insert something you've read]. I am grateful for my glow.

Daily Shit: Reflections about Today's Goals and Outcomes

I'm the **SHIT** because:

I am proud of this because:

This is how I am going to build on that:

Today's **BULLSHIT** is this:

I feel frustrated, disappointed, angry, discouraged

[insert appropriate feeling here]

because:

Here is my solution to this bullshit:

Day 5
Week 3

A DIRTY WORD

"Whatever is bringing you down, get rid of it. Because you'll find that when you're free ... your true self comes out."

-Tina Turner

Today's goals...

Habit	Goals	Outcomes
Sleep		
Water		
Food		
Fitness		
Steps		
Stress		
Habit: ______________		
Habit: ______________		
Habit: ______________		

A MOMENT OF GRATITUDE

When I removed

____

[insert the obstacle, baggage, or burden], I discovered my true self. I am grateful that I freed myself to make that discovery.

Daily Shit: Reflections about Today's Goals and Outcomes

I'm the **SHIT** because:

I am proud of this because:

This is how I am going to build on that:

Today's **BULLSHIT** is this:

I feel frustrated, disappointed, angry, discouraged

[insert appropriate feeling here]

because:

Here is my solution to this bullshit:

Day 6
Week 3

A DIRTY WORD

"I had to make my own living and my own opportunity. But I made it! Don't sit down and wait for the opportunities to come. Get up and make them."

~Madam w. Walker

Today's goals...

Habit	Goals	Outcomes
Sleep		
Water		
Food		
Fitness		
Steps		
Stress		
Habit: ______________		
Habit: ______________		
Habit: ______________		

A MOMENT OF GRATITUDE

I am grateful that I didn't wait for this opportunity to come

____

[insert the opportunity] I made it happen.

Daily Shit: Reflections about Today's Goals and Outcomes

I'm the **SHIT** because:

I am proud of this because:

This is how I am going to build on that:

Today's **BULLSHIT** is this:

I feel frustrated, disappointed, angry, discouraged

[insert appropriate feeling here]

because:

Here is my solution to this bullshit:

Day 7
Week 3

A DIRTY WORD

"The best way to make dreams come true is to wake up."

~Mae C. Jemison

Today's goals...

Habit	Goals	Outcomes
Sleep		
Water		
Food		
Fitness		
Steps		
Stress		
Habit: ____________		
Habit: ____________		
Habit: ____________		

A MOMENT OF GRATITUDE

I am grateful that I didn't keep dreaming about

[insert your response] I woke up, put a plan in place, and followed through with it.

Daily Shit: Reflections about Today's Goals and Outcomes

I'm the **SHIT** because:

I am proud of this because:

This is how I am going to build on that:

Today's **BULLSHIT** is this:

I feel frustrated, disappointed, angry, discouraged

[insert appropriate feeling here]

because:

Here is my solution to this bullshit:

THE WEEKLY TEA ... SPILL IT

What are you most proud of this week?

What challenged you this week?

What lessons will you take with you into next week?

Week 4

Minding My Weekly Business

Crystal ball, what does my upcoming week look like? (choose up to two):

❍ In these streets, on these interstates—everywhere but home

❍ Recommitting to my health and wellness goals—getting back on plan

❍ You know the routine

❍ A schedule that is super crazy

❍ Me time that doesn't include working on my plan

❍ Approaching goal or milestone

❍ My cycle is coming/I'm on my cycle

❍ I am living with the symptoms of perimenopause/menopause.

❍ ______________________________

Now that I have stared into my future, I will commit to focusing on the following (choose up to two):

❍ Meal and snack prep

❍ A mindset that leads me to success

❍ Spice up my routine

❍ Stay calm, stay focused, stay relaxed

❍ Mindful eating in these streets, on these interstates

❍ Meet my sleep goals

❍ Move my body more

❍ Eat within calorie/points budget

❍ Avoid self-sabotage

❍ Manage triggers

❍ Stay in community, attend meetings, get coaching

❍ Manage the symptoms associated with my cycle

❍ Meet myself where I am in this new season of life

❍ ______________________________

This week, my support includes:

____

____

Weekly Preview

Rosenberg Self-Esteem Scale (Rosenberg-SES)

Below is a list of statements dealing with your general feelings about yourself.
Complete these questions based upon your feelings.

1.	On the whole, I am satisfied with myself.
2.	*At times, I think I am no good at all.
3.	I feel that I have a number of good qualities.
4.	I am able to do things as well as most other people.
5.	*I feel I do not have much to be proud of.
6.	*I certainly feel useless at times.
7.	I feel that I'm a person of worth, at least on an equal plane with others.
8.	*I wish I could have more respect for myself.
9.	*All in all, I am inclined to feel that I am a failure.
10.	I take a positive attitude toward myself.

Scoring

Strongly agree = 3;
Agree = 2;
Disagree = 1;
Strongly disagree = 0.
*Items with an asterisk are reverse scored. To calculate the total self-esteem score, sum the scores for the 10 items. The higher the score, the higher the self-esteem.

Score	Level of Self Esteem
0-10	Low
11-20	Moderate
21-30	High

©The Morris Rosenberg Foundation; c/o Department of Sociology; University of Maryland; 2112 Art/Soc Building; College Park, MD 20742-1315

	Strongly Disagree	Disagree	Agree	Strongly Agree

Weekly Goals

This graph is designed to help you create a snapshot of what you hope to accomplish that week.

Focus	**Sun.**	**Mon.**	**Tues.**	
Physical				
Mental				
Emotional				
Spiritual				
Self Care				
Breakfast				
Lunch				
Dinner				
Snacks				

	Wed.	Thurs.	Fri.	Sat.

Day 1
Week 4

A DIRTY WORD

"I realized that beauty was not a thing that I could acquire or consume, it was something I just had to be."

-Lupita Nyong'o

Today's goals...

Habit	Goals	Outcomes
Sleep		
Water		
Food		
Fitness		
Steps		
Stress		
Habit: ____________		
Habit: ____________		
Habit: ____________		

A MOMENT OF GRATITUDE

I am grateful for having the freedom to BE beautiful, to accept and own my entire existence as beautiful. I do this by

____

[insert the obstacle, baggage, or burden].

Daily Shit: Reflections about Today's Goals and Outcomes

I'm the **SHIT** because:

I am proud of this because:

This is how I am going to build on that:

Today's **BULLSHIT** is this:

I feel frustrated, disappointed, angry, discouraged

[insert appropriate feeling here]

because:

Here is my solution to this bullshit:

Day 2
Week 4

A DIRTY WORD

"We have been raised to fear the yes within ourselves, our deepest cravings."
~Audre Lorde

Today's goals...

Habit	Goals	Outcomes
Sleep		
Water		
Food		
Fitness		
Steps		
Stress		
Habit: ______________		
Habit: ______________		
Habit: ______________		

A MOMENT OF GRATITUDE

I own my deepest cravings, my biggest yesses, this includes

____

[insert a desire you have fulfilled]. I'm grateful for these.

Daily Shit: Reflections about Today's Goals and Outcomes

I'm the **SHIT** because:

I am proud of this because:

This is how I am going to build on that:

Today's **BULLSHIT** is this:

I feel frustrated, disappointed, angry, discouraged

[insert appropriate feeling here]

because:

Here is my solution to this bullshit:

Day 3
Week 4

A DIRTY WORD

"Ask for what you want and be prepared to get it!" -Maya Angelou

Today's goals...

Habit	Goals	Outcomes
Sleep		
Water		
Food		
Fitness		
Steps		
Stress		
Habit: ______________		
Habit: ______________		
Habit: ______________		

A MOMENT OF GRATITUDE

I am grateful that I not only have the courage to ask for

____

[insert the thing, person, or experience you want]. I completely embrace the fulfillment of that request.

QUIET AS KEPT

"As women, many of us are conditioned early on to ignore or second guess our intuition which lives in our gut. Whether it's our need for healthy emotional release, choice of food, choice of company, artistic expression, play interests, attire, pain experience, and more. Prioritize your gut! Lean into your intuitive nature. Take cues from your body to discern your needs for rest, movement, nutrition, sensory activation, or withdrawal, and act on them unapologetically."

-Keena Atkinson, R'oujie Wellness, Madison WI

Daily Shit: Reflections about Today's Goals and Outcomes

I'm the **SHIT** because:

I am proud of this because:

This is how I am going to build on that:

Today's **BULLSHIT** is this:

I feel frustrated, disappointed, angry, discouraged

[insert appropriate feeling here]

because:

Here is my solution to this bullshit:

Day 4
Week 4

A DIRTY WORD

"I had chosen freedom, with all its insecurities, and nothing in the world would make me turn away from it."

-Lawrence Hill, author of *Someone Knows My Name*

Today's goals...

Habit	Goals	Outcomes
Sleep		
Water		
Food		
Fitness		
Steps		
Stress		
Habit: ____________		
Habit: ____________		
Habit: ____________		

A MOMENT OF GRATITUDE

I chose freedom, with all its insecurities and stayed the course when so many distractions tried to convince me that bondage was much better. Because of that choice, I am

____

[insert how you are free today]. I am grateful.

Daily Shit: Reflections about Today's Goals and Outcomes

I'm the **SHIT** because:

I am proud of this because:

This is how I am going to build on that:

Today's **BULLSHIT** is this:

I feel frustrated, disappointed, angry, discouraged

[insert appropriate feeling here]

because:

Here is my solution to this bullshit:

Day 5
Week 4

A DIRTY WORD

"If I didn't define myself for myself, I would be crunched into other people's fantasies for me and eaten alive."

-Audre Lorde

Today's goals...

Habit	Goals	Outcomes
Sleep		
Water		
Food		
Fitness		
Steps		
Stress		
Habit: ______________		
Habit: ______________		
Habit: ______________		

A MOMENT OF GRATITUDE

I refused to be "crunched into other people's fantasies for me and eaten alive." I defined myself for myself, and I determined that I would be

____

[insert your definition of yourself]. For this, I am grateful.

Daily Shit: Reflections about Today's Goals and Outcomes

I'm the **SHIT** because:

I am proud of this because:

This is how I am going to build on that:

Today's **BULLSHIT** is this:

I feel frustrated, disappointed, angry, discouraged

[insert appropriate feeling here]

because:

Here is my solution to this bullshit:

Day 6
Week 4

A DIRTY WORD

"We prefer to explore the universe by traveling inward, as opposed to outward."

-Nnedi Okorafor, author of *Binti*

Today's goals...

Habit	Goals	Outcomes
Sleep		
Water		
Food		
Fitness		
Steps		
Stress		
Habit: ______________		
Habit: ______________		
Habit: ______________		

A MOMENT OF GRATITUDE

I am grateful that I am confident enough to explore the universe within me, overlooking the distractions of the outside world. In doing so, within me, I have discovered

____

[insert discovery], and this has been a major key to my freedom.

Daily Shit: Reflections about Today's Goals and Outcomes

I'm the **SHIT** because:

I am proud of this because:

This is how I am going to build on that:

Today's **BULLSHIT** is this:

I feel frustrated, disappointed, angry, discouraged

[insert appropriate feeling here]

because:

Here is my solution to this bullshit:

Day 7
Week 4

A DIRTY WORD

"Them that's got shall get, them that's not shall lose. So the Bible says, and it still is news. Mama may have, Papa may have, but God bless the child that's got his own."
-Billie Holiday

Today's goals...

Habit	Goals	Outcomes
Sleep		
Water		
Food		
Fitness		
Steps		
Stress		
Habit: ____________		
Habit: ____________		
Habit: ____________		

A MOMENT OF GRATITUDE

I am grateful that I got

____

[insert something that you acquired], because it sets me up to keep getting.

Daily Shit: Reflections about Today's Goals and Outcomes

I'm the **SHIT** because:

I am proud of this because:

This is how I am going to build on that:

Today's **BULLSHIT** is this:

I feel frustrated, disappointed, angry, discouraged

[insert appropriate feeling here]

because:

Here is my solution to this bullshit:

THE WEEKLY TEA ... SPILL IT

What are you most proud of this week?

What challenged you this week?

What lessons will you take with you into next week?

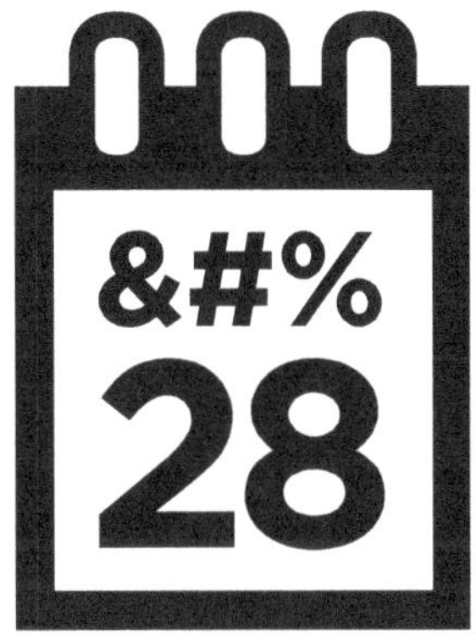

Monthly Shit

You made it through 28 days!
Let's check in using the self-confidence and
self-value exercises that follow.

Self-Value Tank

At the top of each tank, please write a value that you have worked to honor over the past four weeks. For example, you may indicate prayer, good sleep hygiene or healthy touch. Next, indicate how much energy you've put into that value by coloring or shading in the corresponding amount of "gas" you've poured into that particular tank.

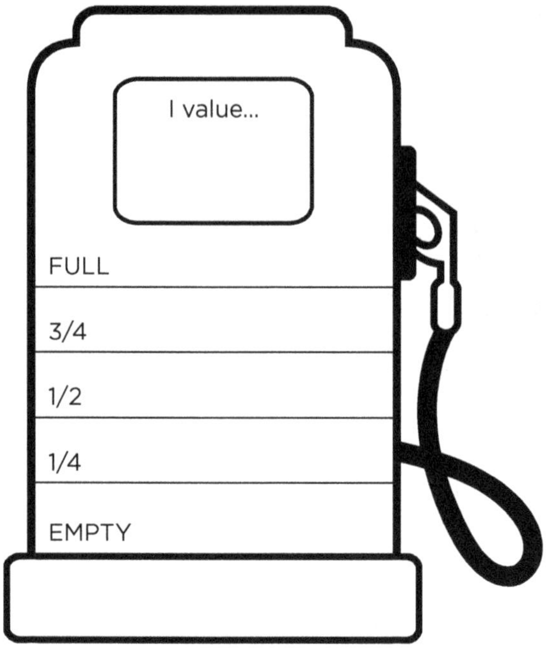

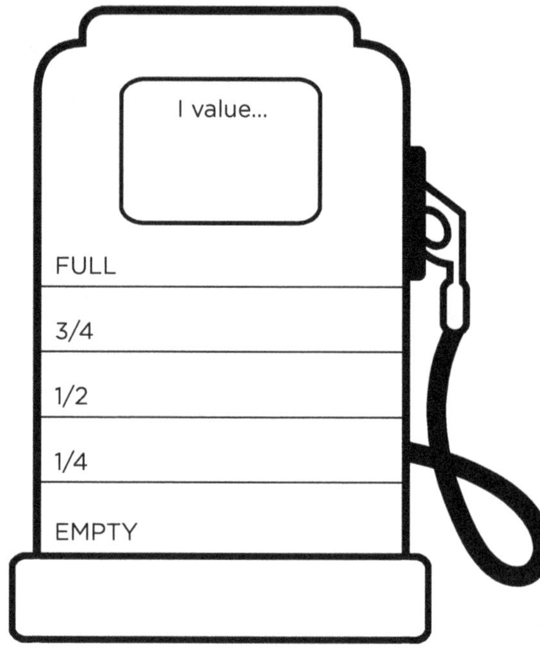

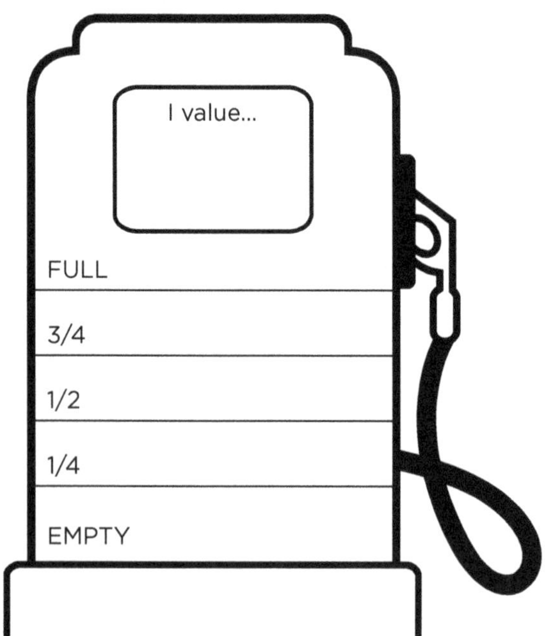

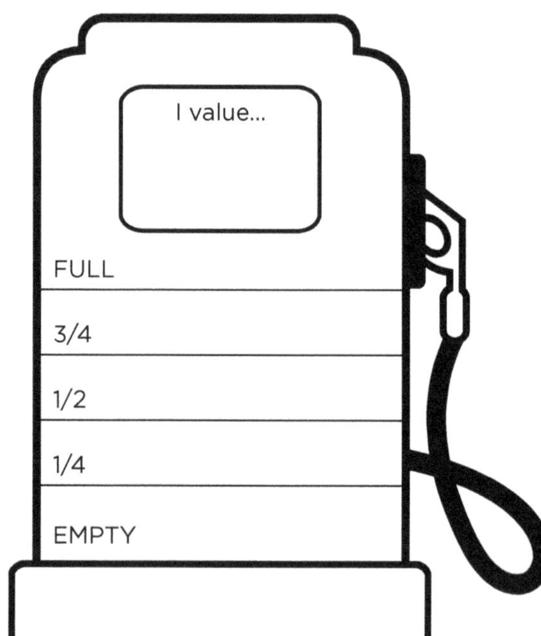

Self-Value Tank Reflection

Self-Confidence Scale

At the end of every month, you will be asked to fill in the layers based on how you are feeling that day and the level of trust have in your ability to overcome your current challenges.

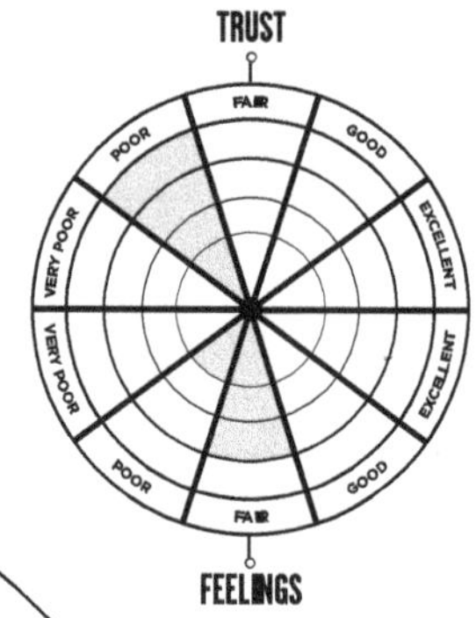

Do you trust yourself to meet your health and wellness goals?

Do you feel that you can meet your health and wellness goals?

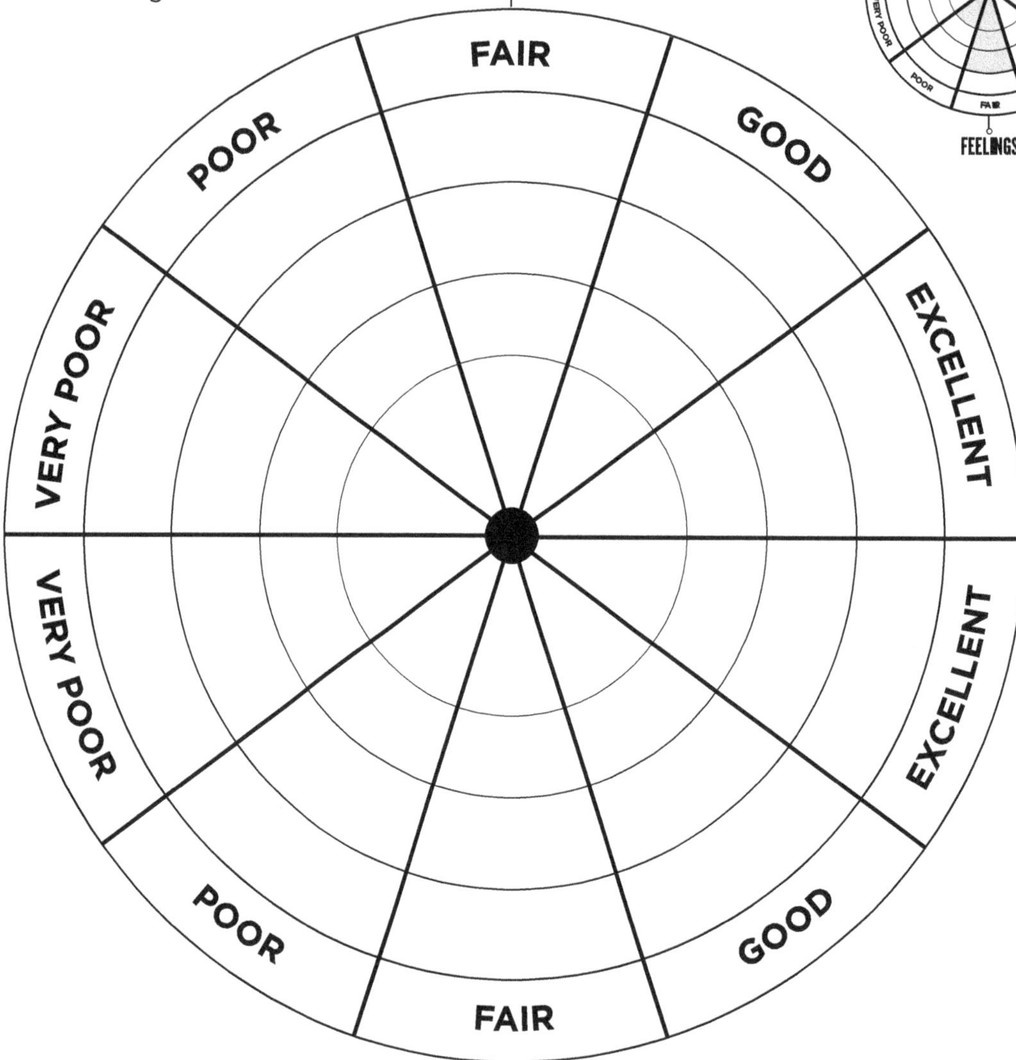

Self-Confidence Scale Reflection

Self-Value

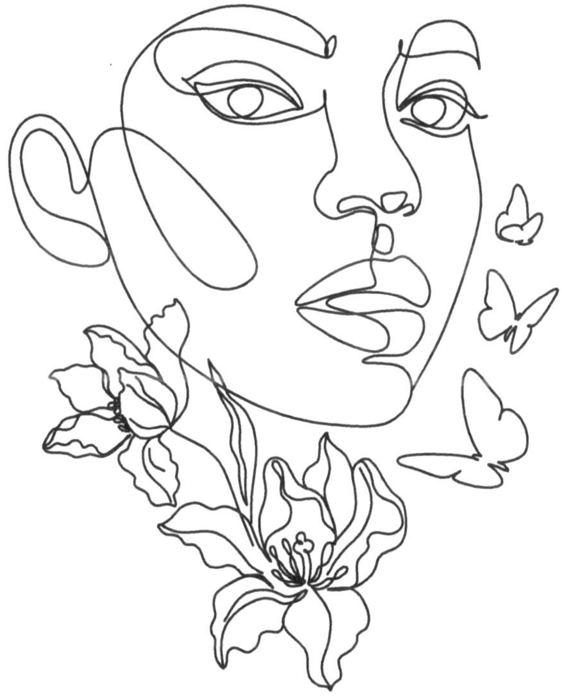

"I am a feminist, and what that means to me is much the same as the meaning of the fact that I am Black; it means that I must undertake to love myself and to respect myself as though my very life depends upon self-love and self-respect."

~June Jordan

Weeks 5-8

Week 5

Minding My Weekly Business

Crystal ball, what does my upcoming week look like? (choose up to two):

❍ In these streets, on these interstates—everywhere but home

❍ Recommitting to my health and wellness goals—getting back on plan

❍ You know the routine

❍ A schedule that is super crazy

❍ Me time that doesn't include working on my plan

❍ Approaching goal or milestone

❍ My cycle is coming/I'm on my cycle

❍ I am living with the symptoms of perimenopause/menopause.

❍ ____________________

Now that I have stared into my future, I will commit to focusing on the following (choose up to two):

❍ Meal and snack prep

❍ A mindset that leads me to success

❍ Spice up my routine

❍ Stay calm, stay focused, stay relaxed

❍ Mindful eating in these streets, on these interstates

❍ Meet my sleep goals

❍ Move my body more

❍ Eat within calorie/points budget

❍ Avoid self-sabotage

❍ Manage triggers

❍ Stay in community, attend meetings, get coaching

❍ Manage the symptoms associated with my cycle

❍ Meet myself where I am in this new season of life

❍ ____________________

This week, my support includes:

____

____

Weekly Preview

Rosenberg Self-Esteem Scale (Rosenberg-SES)

Below is a list of statements dealing with your general feelings about yourself.

Complete these questions based upon your feelings.

1.	On the whole, I am satisfied with myself.
2.	*At times, I think I am no good at all.
3.	I feel that I have a number of good qualities.
4.	I am able to do things as well as most other people.
5.	*I feel I do not have much to be proud of.
6.	*I certainly feel useless at times.
7.	I feel that I'm a person of worth, at least on an equal plane with others.
8.	*I wish I could have more respect for myself.
9.	*All in all, I am inclined to feel that I am a failure.
10.	I take a positive attitude toward myself.

Scoring

Strongly agree = 3;

Agree = 2;

Disagree = 1;

Strongly disagree = 0.

*Items with an asterisk are reverse scored. To calculate the total self-esteem score, sum the scores for the 10 items. The higher the score, the higher the self-esteem.

Score	Level of Self Esteem
0-10	Low
11-20	Moderate
21-30	High

©The Morris Rosenberg Foundation; c/o Department of Sociology; University of Maryland; 2112 Art/Soc Building; College Park, MD 20742-1315

	Strongly Disagree	Disagree	Agree	Strongly Agree

Weekly Goals

This graph is designed to help you create a snapshot of what you hope to accomplish that week.

Focus	**Sun.**	**Mon.**	**Tues.**	
Physical				
Mental				
Emotional				
Spiritual				
Self Care				
Breakfast				
Lunch				
Dinner				
Snacks				

	Wed.	Thurs.	Fri.	Sat.

Day 1
Week 5

A DIRTY WORD

"Learning how to show up for Sagashus was, and still is, the hardest thing I do daily. It's easier to show up for other people than it is to sit in the uncertainty, messiness, and anxiety of my own stuff. It's hard to take responsibility for my gifts, mistakes and time. And yet, I must build a practice of this each day."
~Dr. Sagashus Levingston

Today's goals...

Habit	Goals	Outcomes
Sleep		
Water		
Food		
Fitness		
Steps		
Stress		
Habit: ______________		
Habit: ______________		
Habit: ______________		

A MOMENT OF GRATITUDE

I am grateful for my ability to take responsibility for my entire life. Today, I take responsibility for

____
[insert a gift of yours],

____
[insert a mistake of yours],

____
[insert something on your schedule]. I am working to build a daily practice of showing up for me.

Daily Shit: Reflections about Today's Goals and Outcomes

I'm the **SHIT** because:

I am proud of this because:

This is how I am going to build on that:

Today's **BULLSHIT** is this:

I feel frustrated, disappointed, angry, discouraged

[insert appropriate feeling here]

because:

Here is my solution to this bullshit:

Day 2
Week 5

A DIRTY WORD

"It's time for you to move, realizing that the thing you are seeking is also seeking you."
~Iyanla Vanzant

Today's goals...

Habit	Goals	Outcomes
Sleep		
Water		
Food		
Fitness		
Steps		
Stress		
Habit: ______________		
Habit: ______________		
Habit: ______________		

A MOMENT OF GRATITUDE

I realize that I am who I've been seeking: a woman who is

____

[insert who you've been seeking]. I am grateful that I am moving toward myself.

Daily Shit: Reflections about Today's Goals and Outcomes

I'm the **SHIT** because:

I am proud of this because:

This is how I am going to build on that:

Today's **BULLSHIT** is this:

I feel frustrated, disappointed, angry, discouraged

[insert appropriate feeling here]

because:

Here is my solution to this bullshit:

Day 3
Week 5

A DIRTY WORD

"Do one thing every day that scares you." ~Eleanor Roosevelt

Today's goals...

Habit	Goals	Outcomes
Sleep		
Water		
Food		
Fitness		
Steps		
Stress		
Habit: ____________		
Habit: ____________		
Habit: ____________		

A MOMENT OF GRATITUDE

I am grateful for daily doses of courage. Each day, I commit to doing one thing that scares me. Today, the scary thing I am doing is

____

[insert the thing, person, or experience you want].

QUIET AS KEPT

"Once I learned the importance of showing up no matter how I was feeling, no matter the defeat of the scale, no matter the shame of overeating and anything else in my mind, I was able to receive the blessings and benefits that were awaiting me."

~Marjorie Ledbetter, Covet member, Arlington, TX

Daily Shit: Reflections about Today's Goals and Outcomes

I'm the **SHIT** because:

I am proud of this because:

This is how I am going to build on that:

Today's **BULLSHIT** is this:

I feel frustrated, disappointed, angry, discouraged

[insert appropriate feeling here]

because:

Here is my solution to this bullshit:

Day 4
Week 5

A DIRTY WORD

"I don't really want to become normal, average, standard. I want merely to gain in strength, in the courage to live out my life more fully, enjoy more, experience more. I want to develop even more original and more unconventional traits." -Anaïs Nin

Today's goals...

Habit	Goals	Outcomes
Sleep		
Water		
Food		
Fitness		
Steps		
Stress		
Habit: ______________		
Habit: ______________		
Habit: ______________		

A MOMENT OF GRATITUDE

I am grateful for these five qualities:

1. ______________
2. ______________
3. ______________
4. ______________
5. ______________

They make me unique.

Daily Shit: Reflections about Today's Goals and Outcomes

I'm the **SHIT** because:

I am proud of this because:

This is how I am going to build on that:

Today's **BULLSHIT** is this:

I feel frustrated, disappointed, angry, discouraged

[insert appropriate feeling here]

because:

Here is my solution to this bullshit:

Day 5
Week 5

A DIRTY WORD

"Life is short, and it's up to you to make it sweet."
~Sadie Delany

Today's goals...

Habit	Goals	Outcomes
Sleep		
Water		
Food		
Fitness		
Steps		
Stress		
Habit: ____________		
Habit: ____________		
Habit: ____________		

A MOMENT OF GRATITUDE

I am grateful that I have the audacity to make my time on this earth sweet by doing the following three things:

1. ____________________

2. ____________________

3. ____________________

[insert three things that you do to make your life sweet].

Daily Shit: Reflections about Today's Goals and Outcomes

I'm the **SHIT** because:

I am proud of this because:

This is how I am going to build on that:

Today's **BULLSHIT** is this:

I feel frustrated, disappointed, angry, discouraged

[insert appropriate feeling here]

because:

Here is my solution to this bullshit:

Day 6
Week 5

A DIRTY WORD

"If you prioritize yourself, you are going to save yourself."
~Gabrielle Union

Today's goals...

Habit	Goals	Outcomes
Sleep		
Water		
Food		
Fitness		
Steps		
Stress		
Habit: ________		
Habit: ________		
Habit: ________		

A MOMENT OF GRATITUDE

I prioritize myself by doing these three things

1. ______________________

2. ______________________

3. ______________________

[insert three ways you priortize yourself]. This is how I save myself, and I'm grateful for that.

Daily Shit: Reflections about Today's Goals and Outcomes

I'm the **SHIT** because:

I am proud of this because:

This is how I am going to build on that:

Today's **BULLSHIT** is this:

I feel frustrated, disappointed, angry, discouraged

[insert appropriate feeling here]

because:

Here is my solution to this bullshit:

Day 7
Week 5

A DIRTY WORD

"Your willingness to look at your darkness is what empowers you to change."
~Iyanla Vanzant

Today's goals...

Habit	Goals	Outcomes
Sleep		
Water		
Food		
Fitness		
Steps		
Stress		
Habit: ____________		
Habit: ____________		
Habit: ____________		

A MOMENT OF GRATITUDE

I left this part of myself unexplored

____

[insert your response]. I am willing to look at that now, and in doing so, I am empowered to grow. I'm grateful for that.

Daily Shit: Reflections about Today's Goals and Outcomes

I'm the **SHIT** because:

I am proud of this because:

This is how I am going to build on that:

Today's **BULLSHIT** is this:

I feel frustrated, disappointed, angry, discouraged

[insert appropriate feeling here]

because:

Here is my solution to this bullshit:

THE WEEKLY TEA ... SPILL IT

What are you most proud of this week?

What challenged you this week?

What lessons will you take with you into next week?

Week 6

Minding My Weekly Business

Crystal ball, what does my upcoming week look like? (choose up to two):

❍ In these streets, on these interstates—everywhere but home

❍ Recommitting to my health and wellness goals—getting back on plan

❍ You know the routine

❍ A schedule that is super crazy

❍ Me time that doesn't include working on my plan

❍ Approaching goal or milestone

❍ My cycle is coming/I'm on my cycle

❍ I am living with the symptoms of perimenopause/menopause.

❍ ______________________________

Now that I have stared into my future, I will commit to focusing on the following (choose up to two):

❍ Meal and snack prep

❍ A mindset that leads me to success

❍ Spice up my routine

❍ Stay calm, stay focused, stay relaxed

❍ Mindful eating in these streets, on these interstates

❍ Meet my sleep goals

❍ Move my body more

❍ Eat within calorie/points budget

❍ Avoid self-sabotage

❍ Manage triggers

❍ Stay in community, attend meetings, get coaching

❍ Manage the symptoms associated with my cycle

❍ Meet myself where I am in this new season of life

❍ ______________________________

This week, my support includes:

______________________________ ______________________________

____

Weekly Preview

Rosenberg Self-Esteem Scale (Rosenberg-SES)

Below is a list of statements dealing with your general feelings about yourself.

Complete these questions based upon your feelings.

1.	On the whole, I am satisfied with myself.
2.	*At times, I think I am no good at all.
3.	I feel that I have a number of good qualities.
4.	I am able to do things as well as most other people.
5.	*I feel I do not have much to be proud of.
6.	*I certainly feel useless at times.
7.	I feel that I'm a person of worth, at least on an equal plane with others.
8.	*I wish I could have more respect for myself.
9.	*All in all, I am inclined to feel that I am a failure.
10.	I take a positive attitude toward myself.

Scoring

Strongly agree = 3;

Agree = 2;

Disagree = 1;

Strongly disagree = 0.

*Items with an asterisk are reverse scored. To calculate the total self-esteem score, sum the scores for the 10 items. The higher the score, the higher the self-esteem.

Score	Level of Self Esteem
0-10	Low
11-20	Moderate
21-30	High

©The Morris Rosenberg Foundation; c/o Department of Sociology; University of Maryland; 2112 Art/Soc Building; College Park, MD 20742-1315

	Strongly Disagree	Disagree	Agree	Strongly Agree

Weekly Goals

This graph is designed to help you create a snapshot of what you hope to accomplish that week.

Focus	**Sun.**	**Mon.**	**Tues.**	
Physical				
Mental				
Emotional				
Spiritual				
Self Care				
Breakfast				
Lunch				
Dinner				
Snacks				

	Wed.	Thurs.	Fri.	Sat.

Day 1
Week 6

A DIRTY WORD

"My mission in life is not merely to survive, but to thrive; and to do so with some passion, some compassion, some humor, and some style."

-Maya Angelou

Today's goals...

Habit	Goals	Outcomes
Sleep		
Water		
Food		
Fitness		
Steps		
Stress		
Habit: ____________		
Habit: ____________		
Habit: ____________		

A MOMENT OF GRATITUDE

I am grateful that I do more than survive; I thrive. This is what that looks like for me:

1. ____________
2. ____________
3. ____________

[insert three examples of how you are thriving in your life].

Daily Shit: Reflections about Today's Goals and Outcomes

I'm the **SHIT** because:

I am proud of this because:

This is how I am going to build on that:

Today's **BULLSHIT** is this:

I feel frustrated, disappointed, angry, discouraged

[insert appropriate feeling here]

because:

Here is my solution to this bullshit:

Day 2
Week 6

A DIRTY WORD

"Deal with yourself as an individual worthy of respect, and make everyone else deal with you the same way."
-Nikki Giovanni

Today's goals...

Habit	Goals	Outcomes
Sleep		
Water		
Food		
Fitness		
Steps		
Stress		
Habit: ____________		
Habit: ____________		
Habit: ____________		

A MOMENT OF GRATITUDE

I deal with myself as an individual worthy of respect. This is what that looks like:

1. ____________

2. ____________

3. ____________

[insert three actions you take to treat yourself as an individual worthy of respect]. It never gets old watching other people treating me the same way. I'm grateful for these experiences.

Daily Shit: Reflections about Today's Goals and Outcomes

I'm the **SHIT** because:

I am proud of this because:

This is how I am going to build on that:

Today's **BULLSHIT** is this:

I feel frustrated, disappointed, angry, discouraged

[insert appropriate feeling here]

because:

Here is my solution to this bullshit:

Day 3
Week 6

A DIRTY WORD

"I am no longer accepting the things I cannot change. I am changing the things I cannot accept."
~Angela Davis

Today's goals...

Habit	Goals	Outcomes
Sleep		
Water		
Food		
Fitness		
Steps		
Stress		
Habit: ____________		
Habit: ____________		
Habit: ____________		

A MOMENT OF GRATITUDE

I am no longer accepting things I cannot change. Instead, I am grateful to be changing the things I cannot accept:

1. ______________________________
2. ______________________________
3. ______________________________

[insert three things you are changing that you cannot accept].

QUIET AS KEPT

"Be honest with yourself and be accountable for your own goals. Even when in the community. Don't be afraid to be a pace setter. If you are good with hitting your water goals or other wellness goals ... don't be afraid to push yourself. You inspire others." ~Tanisha Pyron, CEO/founder of Tanisha Lynn Pyron Creative Photography and Covet member, Kalamazoo, MI

Daily Shit: Reflections about Today's Goals and Outcomes

I'm the **SHIT** because:

I am proud of this because:

This is how I am going to build on that:

Today's **BULLSHIT** is this:

I feel frustrated, disappointed, angry, discouraged

[insert appropriate feeling here]

because:

Here is my solution to this bullshit:

Day 4
Week 6

A DIRTY WORD

"I was built this way for a reason, so I'm going to use it."

~Simone Biles

Today's goals...

Habit	Goals	Outcomes
Sleep		
Water		
Food		
Fitness		
Steps		
Stress		
Habit: ________________		
Habit: ________________		
Habit: ________________		

A MOMENT OF GRATITUDE

I move my body in a way that honors how I am built. I do this by

____

[insert how you move your body to honor the way it is built].

I am grateful for this.

Daily Shit: Reflections about Today's Goals and Outcomes

I'm the **SHIT** because:

I am proud of this because:

This is how I am going to build on that:

Today's **BULLSHIT** is this:

I feel frustrated, disappointed, angry, discouraged

[insert appropriate feeling here]

because:

Here is my solution to this bullshit:

Day 5
Week 6

A DIRTY WORD

"You've got to learn to leave the table when love's no longer being served."
~Nina Simone

Today's goals...

Habit	Goals	Outcomes
Sleep		
Water		
Food		
Fitness		
Steps		
Stress		
Habit: ______________		
Habit: ______________		
Habit: ______________		

A MOMENT OF GRATITUDE

Love was no longer being served when

____

[insert the circumstance, the situation, or event], so I left the table, and I am grateful.

Daily Shit: Reflections about Today's Goals and Outcomes

I'm the **SHIT** because:

I am proud of this because:

This is how I am going to build on that:

Today's **BULLSHIT** is this:

I feel frustrated, disappointed, angry, discouraged

[insert appropriate feeling here]

because:

Here is my solution to this bullshit:

Day 6
Week 6

A DIRTY WORD

"Are you crazy? The last thing you want to do is make a scene."

"Well, I'm gonna make a movie if you don't show me some respect."

~Sister Souljah

Today's goals...

Habit	Goals	Outcomes
Sleep		
Water		
Food		
Fitness		
Steps		
Stress		
Habit: ____________		
Habit: ____________		
Habit: ____________		

A MOMENT OF GRATITUDE

I didn't make a scene when

____

[insert name], disrespected me. I made a movie. I am grateful that I valued myself enough to speak up.

Daily Shit: Reflections about Today's Goals and Outcomes

I'm the **SHIT** because:

I am proud of this because:

This is how I am going to build on that:

Today's **BULLSHIT** is this:

I feel frustrated, disappointed, angry, discouraged

[insert appropriate feeling here]

because:

Here is my solution to this bullshit:

Day 7
Week 6

A DIRTY WORD

"Always be smarter than the people who hire you."

~Lena Horne

Today's goals...

Habit	Goals	Outcomes
Sleep		
Water		
Food		
Fitness		
Steps		
Stress		
Habit: ______________		
Habit: ______________		
Habit: ______________		

A MOMENT OF GRATITUDE

I am grateful that I am an expert on

____

[insert your response]. The people who hire me to provide a service or do a job depend on and appreciate me for being smarter than them in this area.

Daily Shit: Reflections about Today's Goals and Outcomes

I'm the **SHIT** because:

I am proud of this because:

This is how I am going to build on that:

Today's **BULLSHIT** is this:

I feel frustrated, disappointed, angry, discouraged

[insert appropriate feeling here]

because:

Here is my solution to this bullshit:

THE WEEKLY TEA ... SPILL IT

What are you most proud of this week?

What challenged you this week?

What lessons will you take with you into next week?

Week 7

Minding My Weekly Business

Crystal ball, what does my upcoming week look like? (choose up to two):

❍ In these streets, on these interstates—everywhere but home

❍ Recommitting to my health and wellness goals—getting back on plan

❍ You know the routine

❍ A schedule that is super crazy

❍ Me time that doesn't include working on my plan

❍ Approaching goal or milestone

❍ My cycle is coming/I'm on my cycle

❍ I am living with the symptoms of perimenopause/menopause.

❍ ______________________________

Now that I have stared into my future, I will commit to focusing on the following (choose up to two):

❍ Meal and snack prep

❍ A mindset that leads me to success

❍ Spice up my routine

❍ Stay calm, stay focused, stay relaxed

❍ Mindful eating in these streets, on these interstates

❍ Meet my sleep goals

❍ Move my body more

❍ Eat within calorie/points budget

❍ Avoid self-sabotage

❍ Manage triggers

❍ Stay in community, attend meetings, get coaching

❍ Manage the symptoms associated with my cycle

❍ Meet myself where I am in this new season of life

❍ ______________________________

This week, my support includes:

____

____

Weekly Preview

Rosenberg Self-Esteem Scale (Rosenberg-SES)

Below is a list of statements dealing with your general feelings about yourself.
Complete these questions based upon your feelings.

1.	On the whole, I am satisfied with myself.
2.	*At times, I think I am no good at all.
3.	I feel that I have a number of good qualities.
4.	I am able to do things as well as most other people.
5.	*I feel I do not have much to be proud of.
6.	*I certainly feel useless at times.
7.	I feel that I'm a person of worth, at least on an equal plane with others.
8.	*I wish I could have more respect for myself.
9.	*All in all, I am inclined to feel that I am a failure.
10.	I take a positive attitude toward myself.

Scoring

Strongly agree = 3;
Agree = 2;
Disagree = 1;
Strongly disagree = 0.
*Items with an asterisk are reverse scored. To calculate the total self-esteem score, sum the scores for the 10 items. The higher the score, the higher the self-esteem.

Score	Level of Self Esteem
0-10	Low
11-20	Moderate
21-30	High

©The Morris Rosenberg Foundation; c/o Department of Sociology; University of Maryland; 2112 Art/Soc Building; College Park, MD 20742-1315

	Strongly Disagree	Disagree	Agree	Strongly Agree

Weekly Goals

This graph is designed to help you create a snapshot of what you hope to accomplish that week.

Focus	**Sun.**	**Mon.**	**Tues.**
Physical			
Mental			
Emotional			
Spiritual			
Self Care			
Breakfast			
Lunch			
Dinner			
Snacks			

	Wed.	Thurs.	Fri.	Sat.

Day 1
Week 7

A DIRTY WORD

"Never ever accept 'Because you are a woman' as a reason for doing or not doing anything."
~Chimamanda Ngozi Adichie

Today's goals...

Habit	Goals	Outcomes
Sleep		
Water		
Food		
Fitness		
Steps		
Stress		
Habit: ____________		
Habit: ____________		
Habit: ____________		

A MOMENT OF GRATITUDE

I don't accept 'because you are a woman' as a reason for doing

____

[insert action]. And I don't accept it as a reason for not doing

____

[insert action]. Whatever I choose to do (or not do) is consistent with my values and not with what social norms dictate. I'm grateful for that.

Daily Shit: Reflections about Today's Goals and Outcomes

I'm the **SHIT** because:

I am proud of this because:

This is how I am going to build on that:

Today's **BULLSHIT** is this:

I feel frustrated, disappointed, angry, discouraged

[insert appropriate feeling here]

because:

Here is my solution to this bullshit:

Day 2
Week 7

A DIRTY WORD

You have been criticizing yourself for years, and it hasn't worked. Try approving of yourself and see what happens."

~Louise L. Hay

Today's goals...

Habit	Goals	Outcomes
Sleep		
Water		
Food		
Fitness		
Steps		
Stress		
Habit: ____________		
Habit: ____________		
Habit: ____________		

A MOMENT OF GRATITUDE

I am grateful that I am no longer criticizing myself

____

[insert what were once the areas of criticism in your life].

I am approving of myself, and it has made all the difference.

Daily Shit: Reflections about Today's Goals and Outcomes

I'm the **SHIT** because:

I am proud of this because:

This is how I am going to build on that:

Today's **BULLSHIT** is this:

I feel frustrated, disappointed, angry, discouraged

[insert appropriate feeling here]

because:

Here is my solution to this bullshit:

Day 3
Week 7

A DIRTY WORD

"Don't waste your time or your money on cheap shit, baby, 'cause all you'll end up doing is paying for everythang twice."

~Terry McMillan, author of Mama

Today's goals...

Habit	Goals	Outcomes
Sleep		
Water		
Food		
Fitness		
Steps		
Stress		
Habit: ____________		
Habit: ____________		
Habit: ____________		

A MOMENT OF GRATITUDE

I am thankful that I invest in

____

[insert area of your life you've invested in], because it has saved me money and time in the long run.

QUIET AS KEPT

"Today, choose you! Make your health and wellness journey a priority. Be patient with yourself along the journey. Change (and results) doesn't happen overnight."

~Qiana Abanukam, CEO/founder of Village Girl Boutique and Covet member, Madison, WI

Daily Shit: Reflections about Today's Goals and Outcomes

I'm the **SHIT** because:

I am proud of this because:

This is how I am going to build on that:

Today's **BULLSHIT** is this:

I feel frustrated, disappointed, angry, discouraged

[insert appropriate feeling here]

because:

Here is my solution to this bullshit:

Day 4
Week 7

A DIRTY WORD

"Choose yourself. And when you do, people will notice you, and they will choose you over and over again."
-Nely Galán

Today's goals...

Habit	Goals	Outcomes
Sleep		
Water		
Food		
Fitness		
Steps		
Stress		
Habit: ____________		
Habit: ____________		
Habit: ____________		

A MOMENT OF GRATITUDE

I am grateful that I chose myself when

____

[insert the moment when you chose yourself]. Because I did it then,

____

[insert name], is doing it now.

Daily Shit: Reflections about Today's Goals and Outcomes

I'm the **SHIT** because:

I am proud of this because:

This is how I am going to build on that:

Today's **BULLSHIT** is this:

I feel frustrated, disappointed, angry, discouraged

[insert appropriate feeling here]

because:

Here is my solution to this bullshit:

Day 5
Week 7

A DIRTY WORD

"The woman who does not require validation from anyone is the most feared individual on the planet."
~Mohadesa Najumi

Today's goals...

Habit	Goals	Outcomes
Sleep		
Water		
Food		
Fitness		
Steps		
Stress		
Habit: ______________		
Habit: ______________		
Habit: ______________		

A MOMENT OF GRATITUDE

I am grateful that I am a woman who does not require validation in

____

[insert the part of your life thst doesn't require validation].

I know I intimidate people because of this. And that's okay.

Daily Shit: Reflections about Today's Goals and Outcomes

I'm the **SHIT** because:

I am proud of this because:

This is how I am going to build on that:

Today's **BULLSHIT** is this:

I feel frustrated, disappointed, angry, discouraged

[insert appropriate feeling here]

because:

Here is my solution to this bullshit:

Day 6
Week 7

A DIRTY WORD

"YES should feel like the sun."

~Shonda Rhimes

Today's goals...

Habit	Goals	Outcomes
Sleep		
Water		
Food		
Fitness		
Steps		
Stress		
Habit: ________________		
Habit: ________________		
Habit: ________________		

A MOMENT OF GRATITUDE

When I said "yes" to

____

[insert something you said yes to], it actually did feel like the sun.

Daily Shit: Reflections about Today's Goals and Outcomes

I'm the **SHIT** because:

I am proud of this because:

This is how I am going to build on that:

Today's **BULLSHIT** is this:

I feel frustrated, disappointed, angry, discouraged

[insert appropriate feeling here]

because:

Here is my solution to this bullshit:

Day 7
Week 7

A DIRTY WORD

"Know your worth. Then add tax."

~Unknown

Today's goals...

Habit	Goals	Outcomes
Sleep		
Water		
Food		
Fitness		
Steps		
Stress		
Habit: ____________		
Habit: ____________		
Habit: ____________		

A MOMENT OF GRATITUDE

I know the value of my work. That's why I charge

___

[insert amount you charged], for

___

[insert a product or service]. That includes my tax.

Daily Shit: Reflections about Today's Goals and Outcomes

I'm the **SHIT** because:

I am proud of this because:

This is how I am going to build on that:

Today's **BULLSHIT** is this:

I feel frustrated, disappointed, angry, discouraged

[insert appropriate feeling here]

because:

Here is my solution to this bullshit:

THE WEEKLY TEA ... SPILL IT

What are you most proud of this week?

What challenged you this week?

What lessons will you take with you into next week?

Week 8

Minding My Weekly Business

Crystal ball, what does my upcoming week look like? (choose up to two):

❍ In these streets, on these interstates—everywhere but home

❍ Recommitting to my health and wellness goals—getting back on plan

❍ You know the routine

❍ A schedule that is super crazy

❍ Me time that doesn't include working on my plan

❍ Approaching goal or milestone

❍ My cycle is coming/I'm on my cycle

❍ I am living with the symptoms of perimenopause/menopause.

❍ ______________________________

Now that I have stared into my future, I will commit to focusing on the following (choose up to two):

❍ Meal and snack prep

❍ A mindset that leads me to success

❍ Spice up my routine

❍ Stay calm, stay focused, stay relaxed

❍ Mindful eating in these streets, on these interstates

❍ Meet my sleep goals

❍ Move my body more

❍ Eat within calorie/points budget

❍ Avoid self-sabotage

❍ Manage triggers

❍ Stay in community, attend meetings, get coaching

❍ Manage the symptoms associated with my cycle

❍ Meet myself where I am in this new season of life

❍ ______________________________

This week, my support includes:

____

____

Weekly Preview

Rosenberg Self-Esteem Scale (Rosenberg-SES)

Below is a list of statements dealing with your general feelings about yourself.
Complete these questions based upon your feelings.

1.	On the whole, I am satisfied with myself.
2.	*At times, I think I am no good at all.
3.	I feel that I have a number of good qualities.
4.	I am able to do things as well as most other people.
5.	*I feel I do not have much to be proud of.
6.	*I certainly feel useless at times.
7.	I feel that I'm a person of worth, at least on an equal plane with others.
8.	*I wish I could have more respect for myself.
9.	*All in all, I am inclined to feel that I am a failure.
10.	I take a positive attitude toward myself.

Scoring

Strongly agree = 3;
Agree = 2;
Disagree = 1;
Strongly disagree = 0.
*Items with an asterisk are reverse scored. To calculate the total self-esteem score, sum the scores for the 10 items. The higher the score, the higher the self-esteem.

Score	Level of Self Esteem
0-10	Low
11-20	Moderate
21-30	High

©The Morris Rosenberg Foundation; c/o Department of Sociology; University of Maryland; 2112 Art/Soc Building; College Park, MD 20742-1315

	Strongly Disagree	Disagree	Agree	Strongly Agree

Day 1
Week 8

A DIRTY WORD

"They prefer their distractions, dreams, and illusions, never aware of the higher pleasures that are there for those who choose to master themselves and their crafts."

~Robert Greene and 50 Cent, authors of *The 50th Law*

Today's goals...

Habit	Goals	Outcomes
Sleep		
Water		
Food		
Fitness		
Steps		
Stress		
Habit: ____________		
Habit: ____________		
Habit: ____________		

A MOMENT OF GRATITUDE

I choose to master myself and the art of

____

[insert the art or skill], because accomplishing

____

[insert an accomplishment you value] matters to me. I am grateful.

Daily Shit: Reflections about Today's Goals and Outcomes

I'm the **SHIT** because:

I am proud of this because:

This is how I am going to build on that:

Today's **BULLSHIT** is this:

I feel frustrated, disappointed, angry, discouraged

[insert appropriate feeling here]

because:

Here is my solution to this bullshit:

Day 2
Week 8

A DIRTY WORD

"If you want to know how people feel about themselves, look at their bank account. Money is the greatest measurement of your mindset. Wealth is less a matter of circumstance than it is a matter of knowledge and choice."

~Dennis Kimbro

Today's goals...

Habit	Goals	Outcomes
Sleep		
Water		
Food		
Fitness		
Steps		
Stress		
Habit: ______		
Habit: ______		
Habit: ______		

A MOMENT OF GRATITUDE

I choose to gain more knowledge about wealth by

____

[insert your response]. I am grateful.

Daily Shit: Reflections about Today's Goals and Outcomes

I'm the **SHIT** because:

I am proud of this because:

This is how I am going to build on that:

Today's **BULLSHIT** is this:

I feel frustrated, disappointed, angry, discouraged

[insert appropriate feeling here]

because:

Here is my solution to this bullshit:

Day 3
Week 8

A DIRTY WORD

"You will learn that to get to where you've never been before, you must first become uncomfortable with where you are now." -Dr. Avis A. Jones-DeWeever

Today's goals...

Habit	Goals	Outcomes
Sleep		
Water		
Food		
Fitness		
Steps		
Stress		
Habit: ______		
Habit: ______		
Habit: ______		

A MOMENT OF GRATITUDE

In order to get comfortable, I had to get uncomfortable with

______

[insert your response]; I am grateful doing so has taken me to

______

[insert your response here], a place in my life I have never been before. I am grateful for this.

QUIET AS KEPT

"Rather than listening to the prescriptions of others or 'experts' about how you should rest, move your body, eat, and take care of your mental health, listen to your own body, heart, and mind. What makes you feel rested and balanced? What movement feels good in your body? What kind of exercise makes you feel stronger and more empowered? What food makes you feel nourished and whole? What kind of self-care helps you to decompress? Honor the wisdom of your body! You are your own best guide on your wellness journey." -Kelly Fox, yoga instructor, Madison, WI

Daily Shit: Reflections about Today's Goals and Outcomes

I'm the **SHIT** because:

I am proud of this because:

This is how I am going to build on that:

Today's **BULLSHIT** is this:

I feel frustrated, disappointed, angry, discouraged

[insert appropriate feeling here]

because:

Here is my solution to this bullshit:

Day 4
Week 8

A DIRTY WORD

"But if the root was sour, what business did she have up there hacking at a leaf?"
~Gwendolyn Brooks

Today's goals...

Habit	Goals	Outcomes
Sleep		
Water		
Food		
Fitness		
Steps		
Stress		
Habit: ______________		
Habit: ______________		
Habit: ______________		

A MOMENT OF GRATITUDE

I am grateful for getting at the root of this problem

____

[insert response here]. Doing so added to my self-value.

Daily Shit: Reflections about Today's Goals and Outcomes

I'm the **SHIT** because:

I am proud of this because:

This is how I am going to build on that:

Today's **BULLSHIT** is this:

I feel frustrated, disappointed, angry, discouraged

[insert appropriate feeling here]

because:

Here is my solution to this bullshit:

Day 5
Week 8

A DIRTY WORD

"If you are silent about your pain, they'll kill you and say you enjoyed it."
~Zora Neale Hurston

Today's goals...

Habit	Goals	Outcomes
Sleep		
Water		
Food		
Fitness		
Steps		
Stress		
Habit: ______________		
Habit: ______________		
Habit: ______________		

A MOMENT OF GRATITUDE

I am grateful that I was not silent about my pain. I spoke up when

____

[insert a situation or circumstance you spoke up]. Now,

____

[insert name, situation, or circumstance] will not be able to kill me, and I can say I enjoyed it.

Daily Shit: Reflections about Today's Goals and Outcomes

I'm the **SHIT** because:

I am proud of this because:

This is how I am going to build on that:

Today's **BULLSHIT** is this:

I feel frustrated, disappointed, angry, discouraged

[insert appropriate feeling here]

because:

Here is my solution to this bullshit:

Day 6
Week 8

A DIRTY WORD

"And it dawned on me. If my actions are not lining up with what I say I value, then I have to either change what I do or change what I say matters to me."

-Dr. Sagashus Levingston

Today's goals...

Habit	Goals	Outcomes
Sleep		
Water		
Food		
Fitness		
Steps		
Stress		
Habit: ______________		
Habit: ______________		
Habit: ______________		

A MOMENT OF GRATITUDE

I changed

____

[action or behavior] so that my actions could line up with my value,

____

[insert value here]. I'm grateful.

Daily Shit: Reflections about Today's Goals and Outcomes

I'm the **SHIT** because:

I am proud of this because:

This is how I am going to build on that:

Today's **BULLSHIT** is this:

I feel frustrated, disappointed, angry, discouraged

[insert appropriate feeling here]

because:

Here is my solution to this bullshit:

Day 7
Week 8

A DIRTY WORD

"I was tired of living a trashy life. So I stopped dealing in and leaving garbage everywhere."
~Dr. Sagashus Levingston

Today's goals...

Habit	Goals	Outcomes
Sleep		
Water		
Food		
Fitness		
Steps		
Stress		
Habit: ____________		
Habit: ____________		
Habit: ____________		

A MOMENT OF GRATITUDE

Order and peace in my life looks like

____

[insert your response]; I am grateful.

Daily Shit: Reflections about Today's Goals and Outcomes

I'm the **SHIT** because:

I am proud of this because:

This is how I am going to build on that:

Today's **BULLSHIT** is this:

I feel frustrated, disappointed, angry, discouraged

[insert appropriate feeling here]

because:

Here is my solution to this bullshit:

THE WEEKLY TEA ... SPILL IT

What are you most proud of this week?

What challenged you this week?

What lessons will you take with you into next week?

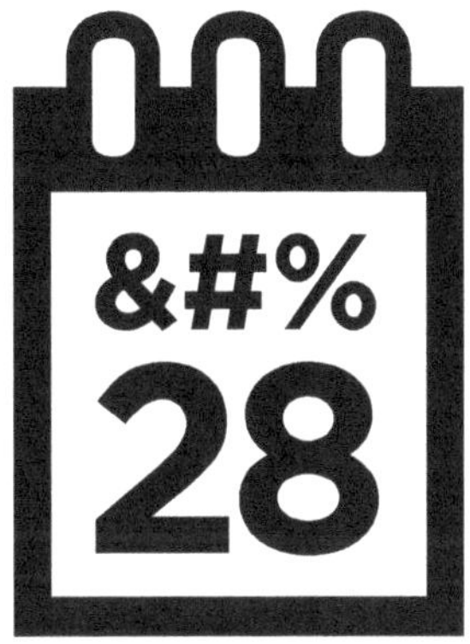

Monthly Shit

You made it through 28 days!
Let's check in using the self-confidence and self-value exercises that follow.

Self-Value Tank

At the top of each tank, please write a value that you have worked to honor over the past four weeks. For example, you may indicate prayer, good sleep hygiene or healthy touch. Next, indicate how much energy you've put into that value by coloring or shading in the corresponding amount of "gas" you've poured into that particular tank.

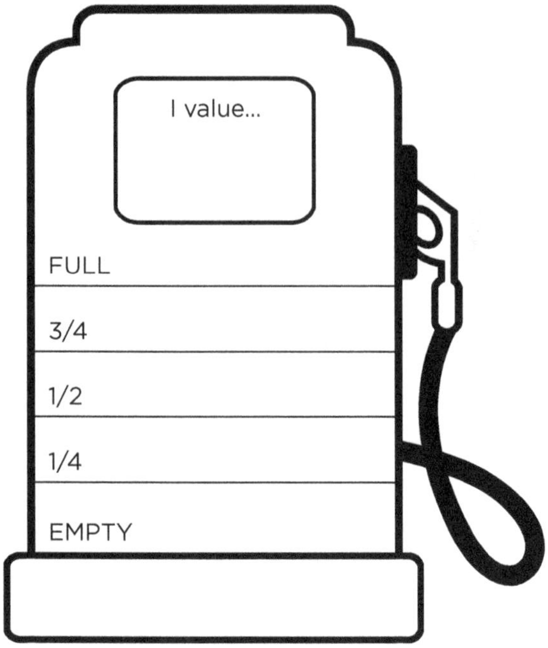

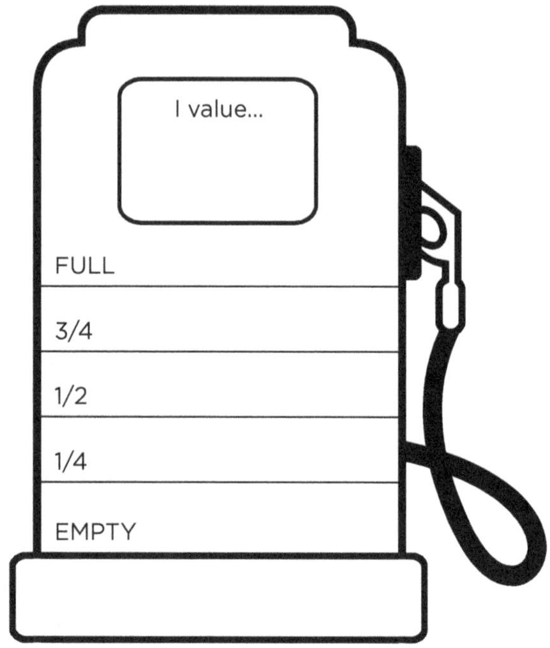

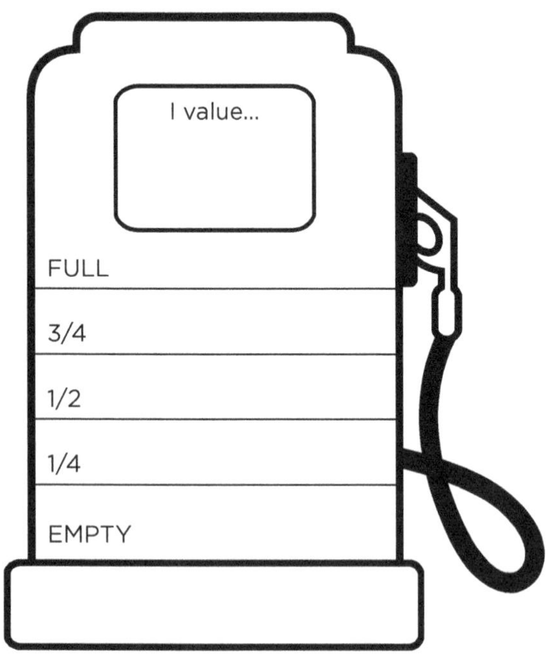

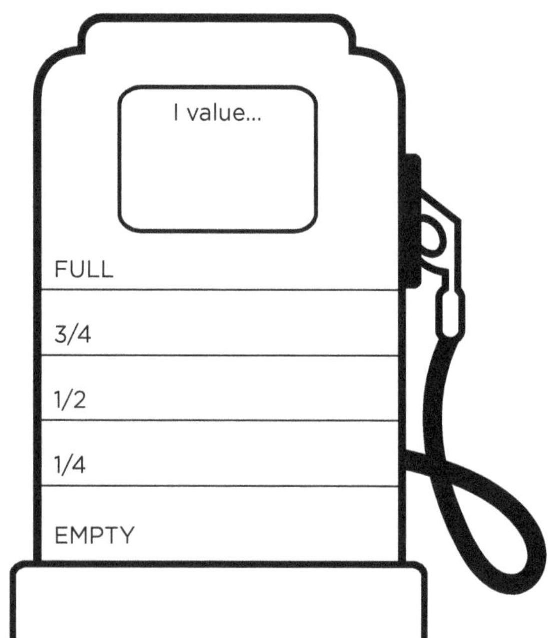

Self-Value Tank Reflection

Self-Confidence Scale

At the end of every month, you will be asked to fill in the layers based on how you are feeling that day and the level of trust have in your ability to overcome your current challenges.

Do you trust yourself to meet your health and wellness goals?

Do you feel that you can meet your health and wellness goals?

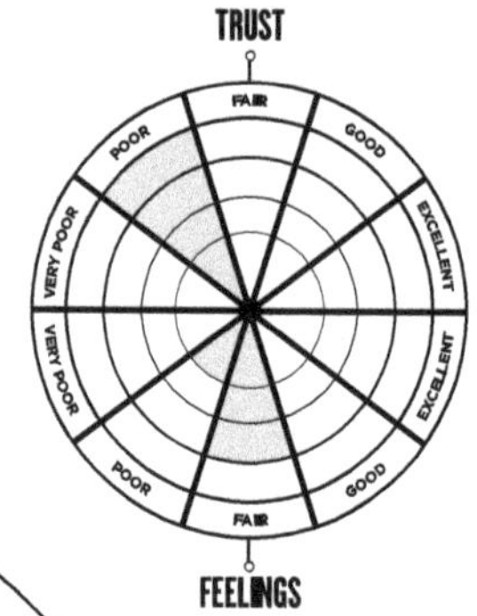

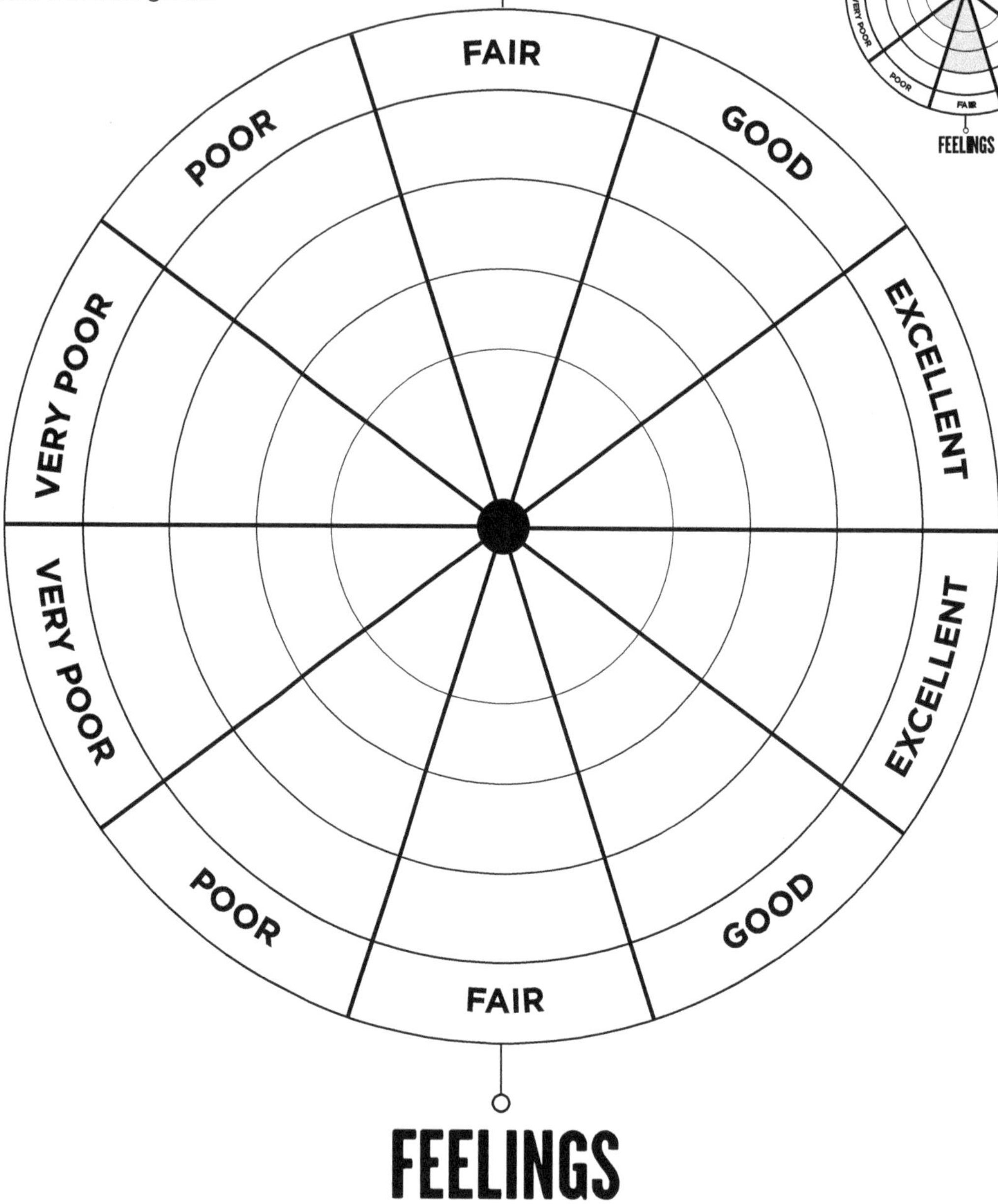

Self-Confidence Scale Reflection

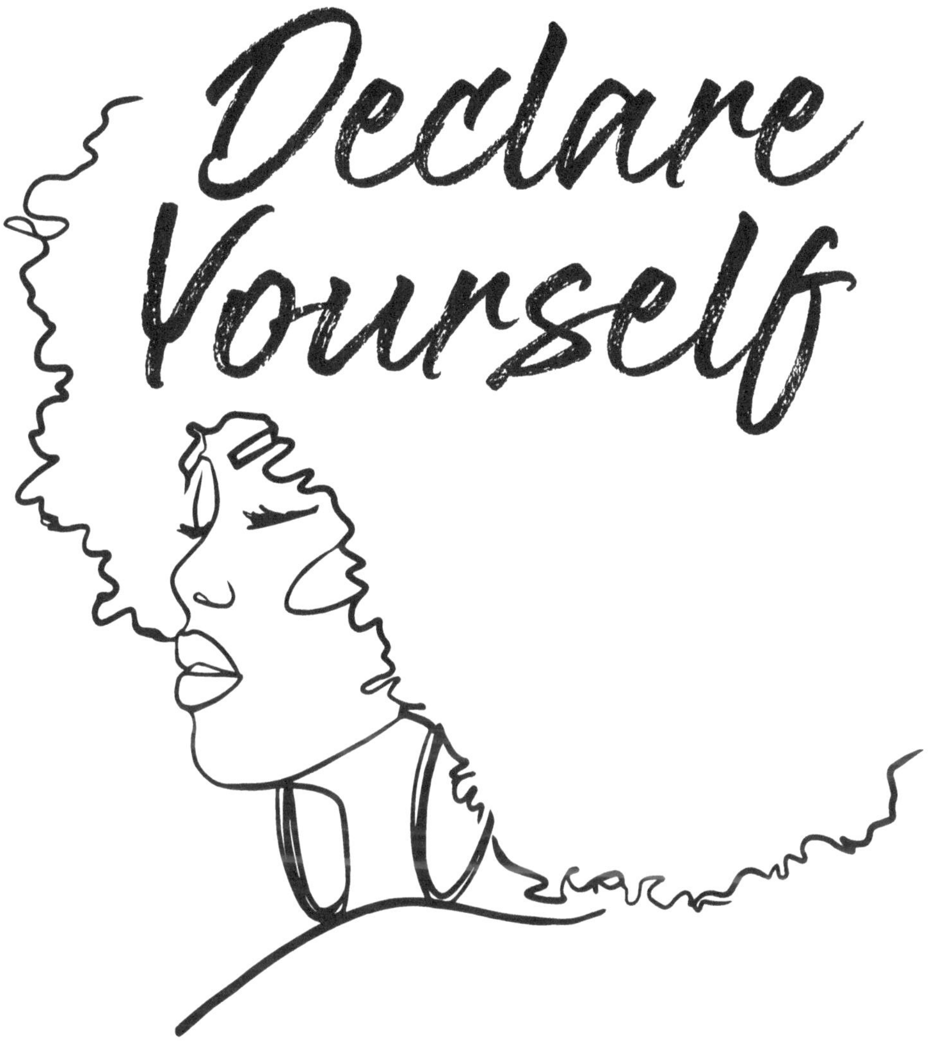

"I am smart, I am talented, I take advantage of the opportunities that come my way and I work really, really hard. Don't call me lucky. Call me a badass."

~Shonda Rhimes

Weeks 9-12

Week 9

Minding My Weekly Business

Crystal ball, what does my upcoming week look like? (choose up to two):

- ❍ In these streets, on these interstates—everywhere but home
- ❍ Recommitting to my health and wellness goals—getting back on plan
- ❍ You know the routine
- ❍ A schedule that is super crazy
- ❍ Me time that doesn't include working on my plan
- ❍ Approaching goal or milestone
- ❍ My cycle is coming/I'm on my cycle
- ❍ I am living with the symptoms of perimenopause/menopause.
- ❍ ______________________________

Now that I have stared into my future, I will commit to focusing on the following (choose up to two):

- ❍ Meal and snack prep
- ❍ A mindset that leads me to success
- ❍ Spice up my routine
- ❍ Stay calm, stay focused, stay relaxed
- ❍ Mindful eating in these streets, on these interstates
- ❍ Meet my sleep goals
- ❍ Move my body more
- ❍ Eat within calorie/points budget
- ❍ Avoid self-sabotage
- ❍ Manage triggers
- ❍ Stay in community, attend meetings, get coaching
- ❍ Manage the symptoms associated with my cycle
- ❍ Meet myself where I am in this new season of life
- ❍ ______________________________

This week, my support includes:

____

____

Weekly Preview

Rosenberg Self-Esteem Scale (Rosenberg-SES)

Below is a list of statements dealing with your general feelings about yourself.
Complete these questions based upon your feelings.

1.	On the whole, I am satisfied with myself.
2.	*At times, I think I am no good at all.
3.	I feel that I have a number of good qualities.
4.	I am able to do things as well as most other people.
5.	*I feel I do not have much to be proud of.
6.	*I certainly feel useless at times.
7.	I feel that I'm a person of worth, at least on an equal plane with others.
8.	*I wish I could have more respect for myself.
9.	*All in all, I am inclined to feel that I am a failure.
10.	I take a positive attitude toward myself.

Scoring

Strongly agree = 3;
Agree = 2;
Disagree = 1;
Strongly disagree = 0.
*Items with an asterisk are reverse scored. To calculate the total self-esteem score, sum the scores for the 10 items. The higher the score, the higher the self-esteem.

Score	Level of Self Esteem
0-10	Low
11-20	Moderate
21-30	High

©The Morris Rosenberg Foundation; c/o Department of Sociology; University of Maryland; 2112 Art/Soc Building; College Park, MD 20742-1315

	Strongly Disagree	Disagree	Agree	Strongly Agree

Weekly Goals

This graph is designed to help you create a snapshot of what you hope to accomplish that week.

Focus	Sun.	Mon.	Tues.	
Physical				
Mental				
Emotional				
Spiritual				
Self Care				
Breakfast				
Lunch				
Dinner				
Snacks				

	Wed.	Thurs.	Fri.	Sat.

Day 1
Week 9

A DIRTY WORD

"Watch as the hood rat messiah climb swiftly
Labels scarred to death to let their artist bomb with me
Cause you can send your thuggest MC and watch me son 'em
The ruggedest bitch, don't even rhyme about gunnin."
~Rah Digga

Today's goals...

Habit	Goals	Outcomes
Sleep		
Water		
Food		
Fitness		
Steps		
Stress		
Habit: ________		
Habit: ________		
Habit: ________		

A MOMENT OF GRATITUDE

I am grateful doing so has taken me to [insert your response]

who saved the day when [insert the ratchet label]

I am that hero no one saw coming [insert the event, circumstance, etc.].

Daily Shit: Reflections about Today's Goals and Outcomes

I'm the **SHIT** because:

I am proud of this because:

This is how I am going to build on that:

Today's **BULLSHIT** is this:

I feel frustrated, disappointed, angry, discouraged

[insert appropriate feeling here]

because:

Here is my solution to this bullshit:

Day 2
Week 9

A DIRTY WORD

"I got a cute face, chubby waist
Thick legs, in shape
Rump shakin' both ways
Make you do a double take
Planet rocker, show stopper
Flow proper, head knocker ..."
~Missy Elliott

Today's goals...

Habit	Goals	Outcomes
Sleep		
Water		
Food		
Fitness		
Steps		
Stress		
Habit: ________________		
Habit: ________________		
Habit: ________________		

A MOMENT OF GRATITUDE

I am grateful that I have a

____

[insert your response]; I am grateful doing so has taken me to

____

[insert adjective] face, [insert adjective] waist,

____

[insert adjective] legs. Make you do a double take.

Daily Shit: Reflections about Today's Goals and Outcomes

I'm the **SHIT** because:

I am proud of this because:

This is how I am going to build on that:

Today's **BULLSHIT** is this:

I feel frustrated, disappointed, angry, discouraged

[insert appropriate feeling here]

because:

Here is my solution to this bullshit:

Day 3
Week 9

A DIRTY WORD

"I can do what you do, easy. Believe me, fronting gives me heebie-jeebies. So while you're imitating Al Capone, I'll be Nina Simone and defecating on your microphone." -Lauryn Hill

Today's goals...

Habit	Goals	Outcomes
Sleep		
Water		
Food		
Fitness		
Steps		
Stress		
Habit: ______		
Habit: ______		
Habit: ______		

A MOMENT OF GRATITUDE

While you're imitating

[insert name], I'll be

[insert name] and

[insert verb] on your

[insert noun]. I'm grateful for my ability to make it look so easy.

QUIET AS KEPT

"Start over as many times as you need to in order to achieve your perfect score."
-Blaq Carrie B, author of *Be Better, Not Bitter*

Daily Shit: Reflections about Today's Goals and Outcomes

I'm the **SHIT** because:

I am proud of this because:

This is how I am going to build on that:

Today's **BULLSHIT** is this:

I feel frustrated, disappointed, angry, discouraged

[insert appropriate feeling here]

because:

Here is my solution to this bullshit:

Day 4
Week 9

A DIRTY WORD

I'm a *Goodfella* kinda lady."

~Lil' Kim

Today's goals...

Habit	Goals	Outcomes
Sleep		
Water		
Food		
Fitness		
Steps		
Stress		
Habit: ____________		
Habit: ____________		
Habit: ____________		

A MOMENT OF GRATITUDE

I am a

____

[insert something really badass and tough] kinda lady. I'm grateful.

Daily Shit: Reflections about Today's Goals and Outcomes

I'm the **SHIT** because:

I am proud of this because:

This is how I am going to build on that:

Today's **BULLSHIT** is this:

I feel frustrated, disappointed, angry, discouraged

[insert appropriate feeling here]

because:

Here is my solution to this bullshit:

Day 5
Week 9

A DIRTY WORD

"I'm a savage (yeah)
Classy, bougie, ratchet (yeah)
Sassy, moody, nasty (hey, hey, yeah)"
~Megan Thee Stallion

Today's goals...

Habit	Goals	Outcomes
Sleep		
Water		
Food		
Fitness		
Steps		
Stress		
Habit: ________________		
Habit: ________________		
Habit: ________________		

A MOMENT OF GRATITUDE

I am a savage:

[Adjective], [adjective], [adjective].

Sassy, [insert an adjective that ends in y],

[insert an adjective that ends in y]. I am grateful for being all of these things.

Daily Shit: Reflections about Today's Goals and Outcomes

I'm the **SHIT** because:

I am proud of this because:

This is how I am going to build on that:

Today's **BULLSHIT** is this:

I feel frustrated, disappointed, angry, discouraged

[insert appropriate feeling here]

because:

Here is my solution to this bullshit:

Day 6
Week 9

A DIRTY WORD

I sat on the throne drinking nectar with Allah.
I got hot and sent an ice age to Europe to cool my thirst.
My oldest daughter is Nefertiti.
The tears from my birth pains created the Nile.
I am a beautiful woman. ~Nikki Giovanni

Today's goals...

Habit	Goals	Outcomes
Sleep		
Water		
Food		
Fitness		
Steps		
Stress		
Habit: ____________		
Habit: ____________		
Habit: ____________		

A MOMENT OF GRATITUDE

I sat on the throne, drinking nectar with

____

[insert the name of someone who is either legendary, mythical or godlike].

____

My oldest child is [insert the name of someone who is either legendary, mythical, or godlike].

____

My birth pains created the [name a body of water]. I am grateful for my power.

____

Daily Shit: Reflections about Today's Goals and Outcomes

I'm the **SHIT** because:

I am proud of this because:

This is how I am going to build on that:

Today's **BULLSHIT** is this:

I feel frustrated, disappointed, angry, discouraged

[insert appropriate feeling here]

because:

Here is my solution to this bullshit:

Day 7
Week 9

A DIRTY WORD

"I just took a DNA test, turns out I'm 100 percent that bitch."
~Lizzo

Today's goals...

Habit	Goals	Outcomes
Sleep		
Water		
Food		
Fitness		
Steps		
Stress		
Habit: ____________		
Habit: ____________		
Habit: ____________		

A MOMENT OF GRATITUDE

I just took a DNA test. Turns out I am 100 percent

____

[insert something sassy and fierce]. I am grateful.

Daily Shit: Reflections about Today's Goals and Outcomes

I'm the **SHIT** because:

I am proud of this because:

This is how I am going to build on that:

Today's **BULLSHIT** is this:

I feel frustrated, disappointed, angry, discouraged

[insert appropriate feeling here]

because:

Here is my solution to this bullshit:

THE WEEKLY TEA ... SPILL IT

What are you most proud of this week?

What challenged you this week?

What lessons will you take with you into next week?

Week 10

Minding My Weekly Business

Crystal ball, what does my upcoming week look like? (choose up to two):

- ❍ In these streets, on these interstates—everywhere but home
- ❍ Recommitting to my health and wellness goals—getting back on plan
- ❍ You know the routine
- ❍ A schedule that is super crazy
- ❍ Me time that doesn't include working on my plan
- ❍ Approaching goal or milestone
- ❍ My cycle is coming/I'm on my cycle
- ❍ I am living with the symptoms of perimenopause/menopause.
- ❍ ______________________________

Now that I have stared into my future, I will commit to focusing on the following (choose up to two):

- ❍ Meal and snack prep
- ❍ A mindset that leads me to success
- ❍ Spice up my routine
- ❍ Stay calm, stay focused, stay relaxed
- ❍ Mindful eating in these streets, on these interstates
- ❍ Meet my sleep goals
- ❍ Move my body more
- ❍ Eat within calorie/points budget
- ❍ Avoid self-sabotage
- ❍ Manage triggers
- ❍ Stay in community, attend meetings, get coaching
- ❍ Manage the symptoms associated with my cycle
- ❍ Meet myself where I am in this new season of life
- ❍ ______________________________

This week, my support includes:

____

____

Weekly Preview

Rosenberg Self-Esteem Scale (Rosenberg-SES)

Below is a list of statements dealing with your general feelings about yourself.

Complete these questions based upon your feelings.

1.	On the whole, I am satisfied with myself.
2.	*At times, I think I am no good at all.
3.	I feel that I have a number of good qualities.
4.	I am able to do things as well as most other people.
5.	*I feel I do not have much to be proud of.
6.	*I certainly feel useless at times.
7.	I feel that I'm a person of worth, at least on an equal plane with others.
8.	*I wish I could have more respect for myself.
9.	*All in all, I am inclined to feel that I am a failure.
10.	I take a positive attitude toward myself.

Scoring

Strongly agree = 3;

Agree = 2;

Disagree = 1;

Strongly disagree = 0.

*Items with an asterisk are reverse scored. To calculate the total self-esteem score, sum the scores for the 10 items. The higher the score, the higher the self-esteem.

Score	Level of Self Esteem
0-10	Low
11-20	Moderate
21-30	High

©The Morris Rosenberg Foundation; c/o Department of Sociology; University of Maryland; 2112 Art/Soc Building; College Park, MD 20742-1315

	Strongly Disagree	Disagree	Agree	Strongly Agree

Weekly Goals

This graph is designed to help you create a snapshot of what you hope to accomplish that week.

Focus	**Sun.**	**Mon.**	**Tues.**	
Physical				
Mental				
Emotional				
Spiritual				
Self Care				
Breakfast				
Lunch				
Dinner				
Snacks				

	Wed.	Thurs.	Fri.	Sat.

Day 1
Week 10

A DIRTY WORD

"I am not a word, I am not a line, I am not a girl that can ever be defined."
~Nicki Minaj

Today's goals...

Habit	Goals	Outcomes
Sleep		
Water		
Food		
Fitness		
Steps		
Stress		
Habit: ______		
Habit: ______		
Habit: ______		

A MOMENT OF GRATITUDE

I am beyond definition. I am neither

[insert response] nor [insert response]. People try to fit me into certain boxes, but they can't. I am grateful for this.

Daily Shit: Reflections about Today's Goals and Outcomes

I'm the **SHIT** because:

I am proud of this because:

This is how I am going to build on that:

Today's **BULLSHIT** is this:

I feel frustrated, disappointed, angry, discouraged

[insert appropriate feeling here]

because:

Here is my solution to this bullshit:

Day 2
Week 10

A DIRTY WORD

"I'm a boss in a skirt, I'm a dog, I'm a flirt."

~Cardi B

Today's goals...

Habit	Goals	Outcomes
Sleep		
Water		
Food		
Fitness		
Steps		
Stress		
Habit: ______________		
Habit: ______________		
Habit: ______________		

A MOMENT OF GRATITUDE

I'm a boss in a skirt, I'm a

____

[insert animal], I'm a

____

[insert something sexy].

Daily Shit: Reflections about Today's Goals and Outcomes

I'm the **SHIT** because:

I am proud of this because:

This is how I am going to build on that:

Today's **BULLSHIT** is this:

I feel frustrated, disappointed, angry, discouraged

[insert appropriate feeling here]

because:

Here is my solution to this bullshit:

Day 3
Week 10

A DIRTY WORD

"I'm a triple threat." ~Beyonce

Today's goals...

Habit	Goals	Outcomes
Sleep		
Water		
Food		
Fitness		
Steps		
Stress		
Habit: ________________		
Habit: ________________		
Habit: ________________		

A MOMENT OF GRATITUDE

I am grateful that I am a triple threat. I am

[insert first threat],

[insert second threat], and,

[insert third threat]. I use these to,

[insert how you empower yourself with your abilities, qualities, features, etc.]

QUIET AS KEPT

"Once, I was 10 pounds away from my goal. My weight increased a bit. I got so discouraged that I gained 80 more. On this journey, the scale goes up and down. When it's going up, learn to laugh and say, 'You won't get me with that one.' Keep showing up for your goals because if you stick with the plan, eventually, the scale will reflect your efforts. In the meantime, you're creating a lifestyle filled with healthy habits that will change your entire life for the better."
~Dr. Sagashus Levingston, CEO/founder of Infamous Mothers, LLC, Madison, WI

Daily Shit: Reflections about Today's Goals and Outcomes

I'm the **SHIT** because:

I am proud of this because:

This is how I am going to build on that:

Today's **BULLSHIT** is this:

I feel frustrated, disappointed, angry, discouraged

[insert appropriate feeling here]

because:

Here is my solution to this bullshit:

Day 4
Week 10

A DIRTY WORD

"I'm a woman
Phenomenally.
Phenomenal woman,
That's me."
~Maya Angelou

Today's goals...

Habit	Goals	Outcomes
Sleep		
Water		
Food		
Fitness		
Steps		
Stress		
Habit: ______		
Habit: ______		
Habit: ______		

A MOMENT OF GRATITUDE

I am grateful that I am a phenomenal woman.
I am extraordinary in these three ways.

1. ______
2. ______
3. ______

Daily Shit: Reflections about Today's Goals and Outcomes

I'm the **SHIT** because:

I am proud of this because:

This is how I am going to build on that:

Today's **BULLSHIT** is this:

I feel frustrated, disappointed, angry, discouraged

[insert appropriate feeling here]

because:

Here is my solution to this bullshit:

Day 5
Week 10

A DIRTY WORD

"My mother always wanted me to be a jazz singer, but I always wanted to be raunchy."
~Etta James

Today's goals...

Habit	Goals	Outcomes
Sleep		
Water		
Food		
Fitness		
Steps		
Stress		
Habit: __________		
Habit: __________		
Habit: __________		

A MOMENT OF GRATITUDE

My mother wanted me to be a

____

[insert what she wanted you to be]. I am grateful that I became

____

[insert what you became—it has to be something contrary to what your mom wanted].

Daily Shit: Reflections about Today's Goals and Outcomes

I'm the **SHIT** because:

I am proud of this because:

This is how I am going to build on that:

Today's **BULLSHIT** is this:

I feel frustrated, disappointed, angry, discouraged

[insert appropriate feeling here]

because:

Here is my solution to this bullshit:

Day 6
Week 10

A DIRTY WORD

"I am self-made."

-Nely Galán

Today's goals...

Habit	Goals	Outcomes
Sleep		
Water		
Food		
Fitness		
Steps		
Stress		
Habit: ______________		
Habit: ______________		
Habit: ______________		

A MOMENT OF GRATITUDE

I am grateful that I am self-made. It may have taken a village to get me to where I am, but it was my:

____

[insert response] that drove the process.

Daily Shit: Reflections about Today's Goals and Outcomes

I'm the **SHIT** because:

I am proud of this because:

This is how I am going to build on that:

Today's **BULLSHIT** is this:

I feel frustrated, disappointed, angry, discouraged

[insert appropriate feeling here]

because:

Here is my solution to this bullshit:

Day 7
Week 10

A DIRTY WORD

"I'm a dangerous woman."

~Pat Mitchell

Today's goals...

Habit	**Goals**	**Outcomes**
Sleep		
Water		
Food		
Fitness		
Steps		
Stress		
Habit: ________________		
Habit: ________________		
Habit: ________________		

A MOMENT OF GRATITUDE

I am grateful that I am a dangerous woman. I am dangerous because

____

[insert what makes you dangerous].

Daily Shit: Reflections about Today's Goals and Outcomes

I'm the **SHIT** because:

I am proud of this because:

This is how I am going to build on that:

Today's **BULLSHIT** is this:

I feel frustrated, disappointed, angry, discouraged

[insert appropriate feeling here]

because:

Here is my solution to this bullshit:

THE WEEKLY TEA ... SPILL IT

What are you most proud of this week?

What challenged you this week?

What lessons will you take with you into next week?

Week 11

Minding My Weekly Business

Crystal ball, what does my upcoming week look like? (choose up to two):

❍ In these streets, on these interstates—everywhere but home

❍ Recommitting to my health and wellness goals—getting back on plan

❍ You know the routine

❍ A schedule that is super crazy

❍ Me time that doesn't include working on my plan

❍ Approaching goal or milestone

❍ My cycle is coming/I'm on my cycle

❍ I am living with the symptoms of perimenopause/menopause.

❍ ______________________________

Now that I have stared into my future, I will commit to focusing on the following (choose up to two):

❍ Meal and snack prep

❍ A mindset that leads me to success

❍ Spice up my routine

❍ Stay calm, stay focused, stay relaxed

❍ Mindful eating in these streets, on these interstates

❍ Meet my sleep goals

❍ Move my body more

❍ Eat within calorie/points budget

❍ Avoid self-sabotage

❍ Manage triggers

❍ Stay in community, attend meetings, get coaching

❍ Manage the symptoms associated with my cycle

❍ Meet myself where I am in this new season of life

❍ ______________________________

This week, my support includes:

____

____

____

Weekly Preview

Rosenberg Self-Esteem Scale (Rosenberg-SES)

Below is a list of statements dealing with your general feelings about yourself.
Complete these questions based upon your feelings.

1.	On the whole, I am satisfied with myself.
2.	*At times, I think I am no good at all.
3.	I feel that I have a number of good qualities.
4.	I am able to do things as well as most other people.
5.	*I feel I do not have much to be proud of.
6.	*I certainly feel useless at times.
7.	I feel that I'm a person of worth, at least on an equal plane with others.
8.	*I wish I could have more respect for myself.
9.	*All in all, I am inclined to feel that I am a failure.
10.	I take a positive attitude toward myself.

Scoring

Strongly agree = 3;
Agree = 2;
Disagree = 1;
Strongly disagree = 0.
*Items with an asterisk are reverse scored. To calculate the total self-esteem score, sum the scores for the 10 items. The higher the score, the higher the self-esteem.

Score	Level of Self Esteem
0-10	Low
11-20	Moderate
21-30	High

©The Morris Rosenberg Foundation; c/o Department of Sociology; University of Maryland; 2112 Art/Soc Building; College Park, MD 20742-1315

	Strongly Disagree	Disagree	Agree	Strongly Agree

Weekly Goals

This graph is designed to help you create a snapshot of what you hope to accomplish that week.

Focus	**Sun.**	**Mon.**	**Tues.**
Physical			
Mental			
Emotional			
Spiritual			
Self Care			
Breakfast			
Lunch			
Dinner			
Snacks			

	Wed.	Thurs.	Fri.	Sat.

Day 1
Week 11

A DIRTY WORD

"I am Daenerys Stormborn of the House Targaryen, the First of Her Name, the Unburnt, Queen of Meereen, Queen of the Andals and the Rhoynar and the First Men, Khaleesi of the Great Grass Sea, Breaker of Chains and Mother of Dragons."

~Daenerys Targaryen

Today's goals...

Habit	Goals	Outcomes
Sleep		
Water		
Food		
Fitness		
Steps		
Stress		
Habit: ____________		
Habit: ____________		
Habit: ____________		

A MOMENT OF GRATITUDE

I am grateful that I am

[insert your name],

[insert title of choice],

[insert another title of choice],

[insert another title] because [insert your response].

Daily Shit: Reflections about Today's Goals and Outcomes

I'm the **SHIT** because:

I am proud of this because:

This is how I am going to build on that:

Today's **BULLSHIT** is this:

I feel frustrated, disappointed, angry, discouraged

[insert appropriate feeling here]

because:

Here is my solution to this bullshit:

Day 2
Week 11

A DIRTY WORD

"I think I'm the greatest chick in the game, and I expect all the others to feel the same way. If not, you're in the wrong profession."

-Remy Ma

Today's goals...

Habit	Goals	Outcomes
Sleep		
Water		
Food		
Fitness		
Steps		
Stress		
Habit: ____________		
Habit: ____________		
Habit: ____________		

A MOMENT OF GRATITUDE

I am the greatest

____

[insert your response]. I'm grateful.

Daily Shit: Reflections about Today's Goals and Outcomes

I'm the **SHIT** because:

I am proud of this because:

This is how I am going to build on that:

Today's **BULLSHIT** is this:

I feel frustrated, disappointed, angry, discouraged

[insert appropriate feeling here]

because:

Here is my solution to this bullshit:

Day 3
Week 11

A DIRTY WORD

"I can do what you do, easy. Believe me, fronting gives me heebie-jeebies. So while you're imitating Al Capone, I'll be Nina Simone and defecating on your microphone." ~Lauryn Hill

Today's goals...

Habit	Goals	Outcomes
Sleep		
Water		
Food		
Fitness		
Steps		
Stress		
Habit: ______________		
Habit: ______________		
Habit: ______________		

A MOMENT OF GRATITUDE

I am grateful that I am:

____

[insert your name], child of,

____

[insert parent 1's name] and,

____

[insert parent 2's name] because, [insert your response].

QUIET AS KEPT

"Make a playlist of your favorite nasty and/or embarrassing songs you can't play out loud."
~Gretchen Treiber Girard, Madison, WI, Fitness Instructor and Lead Instructor for Covet Fitness

Daily Shit: Reflections about Today's Goals and Outcomes

I'm the **SHIT** because:

I am proud of this because:

This is how I am going to build on that:

Today's **BULLSHIT** is this:

I feel frustrated, disappointed, angry, discouraged

[insert appropriate feeling here]

because:

Here is my solution to this bullshit:

Day 4
Week 11

A DIRTY WORD

"Even if it makes others uncomfortable, I will love who I am."
~Janelle Monáe

Today's goals...

Habit	Goals	Outcomes
Sleep		
Water		
Food		
Fitness		
Steps		
Stress		
Habit: ____________		
Habit: ____________		
Habit: ____________		

A MOMENT OF GRATITUDE

Even if it makes others uncomfortable, I will love being

____

[insert your response]. I am grateful for living out loud.

Daily Shit: Reflections about Today's Goals and Outcomes

I'm the **SHIT** because:

I am proud of this because:

This is how I am going to build on that:

Today's **BULLSHIT** is this:

I feel frustrated, disappointed, angry, discouraged

[insert appropriate feeling here]

because:

Here is my solution to this bullshit:

Day 5
Week 11

A DIRTY WORD

"On an ordinary day, I am a shapeshifter, a seer ... a conjure woman. But when I'm really feeling myself, I tell people, 'I am a CEO, founder, author, and single mother of six.'"
-Dr. Sagashus Levingston

Today's goals...

Habit	Goals	Outcomes
Sleep		
Water		
Food		
Fitness		
Steps		
Stress		
Habit: ____________		
Habit: ____________		
Habit: ____________		

A MOMENT OF GRATITUDE

On an ordinary day, I am a

[insert something mythical], a

[insert something taboo]. But when I am really feeling myself, I tell people, "I am a

[insert of title choice] and a mom of: [insert number of children]. I am grateful.

Daily Shit: Reflections about Today's Goals and Outcomes

I'm the **SHIT** because:

I am proud of this because:

This is how I am going to build on that:

Today's **BULLSHIT** is this:

I feel frustrated, disappointed, angry, discouraged

[insert appropriate feeling here]

because:

Here is my solution to this bullshit:

Day 6
Week 11

A DIRTY WORD

"I'm every woman. It's all in me."

~Chaka Khan

Today's goals...

Habit	Goals	Outcomes
Sleep		
Water		
Food		
Fitness		
Steps		
Stress		
Habit: ______________		
Habit: ______________		
Habit: ______________		

A MOMENT OF GRATITUDE

I'm every woman. It's all in me.

1. ______________________________

2. ______________________________

3. ______________________________

[insert three roles you play or "hats" you wear]. I do it naturally. I am grateful.

Daily Shit: Reflections about Today's Goals and Outcomes

I'm the **SHIT** because:

I am proud of this because:

This is how I am going to build on that:

Today's **BULLSHIT** is this:

I feel frustrated, disappointed, angry, discouraged

[insert appropriate feeling here]

because:

Here is my solution to this bullshit:

Day 7
Week 11

A DIRTY WORD

"I live in a queendom, ruled by a womb-iverse."
~Erykah Badu

Today's goals...

Habit	Goals	Outcomes
Sleep		
Water		
Food		
Fitness		
Steps		
Stress		
Habit: ____________		
Habit: ____________		
Habit: ____________		

A MOMENT OF GRATITUDE

I live in a

____

[insert word + "-dom"], ruled by a

____

[insert + "-iverse"]. I'm grateful.

Daily Shit: Reflections about Today's Goals and Outcomes

I'm the **SHIT** because:

I am proud of this because:

This is how I am going to build on that:

Today's **BULLSHIT** is this:

I feel frustrated, disappointed, angry, discouraged

[insert appropriate feeling here]

because:

Here is my solution to this bullshit:

THE WEEKLY TEA ... SPILL IT

What are you most proud of this week?

What challenged you this week?

What lessons will you take with you into next week?

Week 12

Minding My Weekly Business

Crystal ball, what does my upcoming week look like? (choose up to two):

- ❍ In these streets, on these interstates—everywhere but home
- ❍ Recommitting to my health and wellness goals—getting back on plan
- ❍ You know the routine
- ❍ A schedule that is super crazy
- ❍ Me time that doesn't include working on my plan
- ❍ Approaching goal or milestone
- ❍ My cycle is coming/I'm on my cycle
- ❍ I am living with the symptoms of perimenopause/menopause.
- ❍ ______________________________

Now that I have stared into my future, I will commit to focusing on the following (choose up to two):

- ❍ Meal and snack prep
- ❍ A mindset that leads me to success
- ❍ Spice up my routine
- ❍ Stay calm, stay focused, stay relaxed
- ❍ Mindful eating in these streets, on these interstates
- ❍ Meet my sleep goals
- ❍ Move my body more
- ❍ Eat within calorie/points budget
- ❍ Avoid self-sabotage
- ❍ Manage triggers
- ❍ Stay in community, attend meetings, get coaching
- ❍ Manage the symptoms associated with my cycle
- ❍ Meet myself where I am in this new season of life
- ❍ ______________________________

This week, my support includes:

____

____

Weekly Preview

Rosenberg Self-Esteem Scale (Rosenberg-SES)

Below is a list of statements dealing with your general feelings about yourself.
Complete these questions based upon your feelings.

1.	On the whole, I am satisfied with myself.
2.	*At times, I think I am no good at all.
3.	I feel that I have a number of good qualities.
4.	I am able to do things as well as most other people.
5.	*I feel I do not have much to be proud of.
6.	*I certainly feel useless at times.
7.	I feel that I'm a person of worth, at least on an equal plane with others.
8.	*I wish I could have more respect for myself.
9.	*All in all, I am inclined to feel that I am a failure.
10.	I take a positive attitude toward myself.

Scoring

Strongly agree = 3;
Agree = 2;
Disagree = 1;
Strongly disagree = 0.
*Items with an asterisk are reverse scored. To calculate the total self-esteem score, sum the scores for the 10 items. The higher the score, the higher the self-esteem.

Score	Level of Self Esteem
0-10	Low
11-20	Moderate
21-30	High

©The Morris Rosenberg Foundation; c/o Department of Sociology; University of Maryland; 2112 Art/Soc Building; College Park, MD 20742-1315

	Strongly Disagree	Disagree	Agree	Strongly Agree

Weekly Goals

This graph is designed to help you create a snapshot of what you hope to accomplish that week.

Focus	**Sun.**	**Mon.**	**Tues.**	
Physical				
Mental				
Emotional				
Spiritual				
Self Care				
Breakfast				
Lunch				
Dinner				
Snacks				

	Wed.	Thurs.	Fri.	Sat.

Day 1
Week 12

A DIRTY WORD

"'Cause privacy is my middle name
My last name is control.
No, my first name ain't baby.
It's Janet, Miss Jackson if you're nasty."
~Janet Jackson

Today's goals...

Habit	Goals	Outcomes
Sleep		
Water		
Food		
Fitness		
Steps		
Stress		
Habit: ______________		
Habit: ______________		
Habit: ______________		

A MOMENT OF GRATITUDE

'Cause

____

[insert a word for your genitalia] is my middle name. My last name is control.
No, my first name ain't baby. It's

____

[insert your first name],

____

Miss [insert your last name] if you're nasty. I'm grateful.

Daily Shit: Reflections about Today's Goals and Outcomes

I'm the **SHIT** because:

I am proud of this because:

This is how I am going to build on that:

Today's **BULLSHIT** is this:

I feel frustrated, disappointed, angry, discouraged

[insert appropriate feeling here]

because:

Here is my solution to this bullshit:

Day 2
Week 12

A DIRTY WORD

"I'm a bitch, I'm a lover, I'm a child, I'm a mother
I'm a sinner, I'm a saint, I do not feel ashamed
I'm your hell, I'm your dream, I'm nothing in between."
~Alanis Morissette

Today's goals...

Habit	Goals	Outcomes
Sleep		
Water		
Food		
Fitness		
Steps		
Stress		
Habit: ___________		
Habit: ___________		
Habit: ___________		

A MOMENT OF GRATITUDE

I'm a

____

[insert something vulgar or "unlady-like"], I'm a lover, I'm a child, I'm a mother, I'm a sinner, I'm a saint, I do not feel ashamed.

Daily Shit: Reflections about Today's Goals and Outcomes

I'm the **SHIT** because:

I am proud of this because:

This is how I am going to build on that:

Today's **BULLSHIT** is this:

I feel frustrated, disappointed, angry, discouraged

[insert appropriate feeling here]

because:

Here is my solution to this bullshit:

Day 3
Week 12

A DIRTY WORD

"I'm a triple threat." ~Beyonce

Today's goals...

Habit	Goals	Outcomes
Sleep		
Water		
Food		
Fitness		
Steps		
Stress		
Habit: ______		
Habit: ______		
Habit: ______		

A MOMENT OF GRATITUDE

I'm not that

____

[insert adjective] little person still:

____

[insert verb] over/about you. I'm grateful.

QUIET AS KEPT

"Don't let the scale trick you! On this journey, the scale goes up and down. When it's going up, I laugh and say, "You won't get me with that one." And I keep showing up for my goals because I know that if I stick with the plan, eventually, it will reflect my efforts. In the meantime, I'm creating a lifestyle filled with healthy habits, and my entire life has changed for the better because of it. I hope the same for you"

~Dr. Sagashus Levingston, CEO/Founder of Infamous Mothers, Covet Member

Daily Shit: Reflections about Today's Goals and Outcomes

I'm the **SHIT** because:

I am proud of this because:

This is how I am going to build on that:

Today's **BULLSHIT** is this:

I feel frustrated, disappointed, angry, discouraged

[insert appropriate feeling here]

because:

Here is my solution to this bullshit:

Day 4
Week 12

A DIRTY WORD

"I woke up like this."

~Beyonce, "Flawless"

Today's goals...

Habit	Goals	Outcomes
Sleep		
Water		
Food		
Fitness		
Steps		
Stress		
Habit: ____________		
Habit: ____________		
Habit: ____________		

A MOMENT OF GRATITUDE

I woke up

1. ____________

2. ____________

3. ____________

[insert three positive adjectives]. Flawless. I'm grateful.

Daily Shit: Reflections about Today's Goals and Outcomes

I'm the **SHIT** because:

I am proud of this because:

This is how I am going to build on that:

Today's **BULLSHIT** is this:

I feel frustrated, disappointed, angry, discouraged

[insert appropriate feeling here]

because:

Here is my solution to this bullshit:

Day 5
Week 12

A DIRTY WORD

"Sis, becoming a Black Woman Millionaire is a revolutionary act."
~Dr. Venus Opal Reese

Today's goals...

Habit	Goals	Outcomes
Sleep		
Water		
Food		
Fitness		
Steps		
Stress		
Habit: ____________		
Habit: ____________		
Habit: ____________		

A MOMENT OF GRATITUDE

Becoming a mom who is a(n)

____

[insert something far-fetched or impossible] is a revolutionary act.
I am grateful to be aspiring toward this goal.

Daily Shit: Reflections about Today's Goals and Outcomes

I'm the **SHIT** because:

I am proud of this because:

This is how I am going to build on that:

Today's **BULLSHIT** is this:

I feel frustrated, disappointed, angry, discouraged

[insert appropriate feeling here]

because:

Here is my solution to this bullshit:

Day 6
Week 12

A DIRTY WORD

I gotta fly, I need a jet, shit
I need room for my legs.
~Cardi B

Today's goals...

Habit	Goals	Outcomes
Sleep		
Water		
Food		
Fitness		
Steps		
Stress		
Habit: ______________		
Habit: ______________		
Habit: ______________		

A MOMENT OF GRATITUDE

I gotta fly, I need

____

[insert noun], shit. I need room for my

____

[insert body part(s)].

Daily Shit: Reflections about Today's Goals and Outcomes

I'm the **SHIT** because:

I am proud of this because:

This is how I am going to build on that:

Today's **BULLSHIT** is this:

I feel frustrated, disappointed, angry, discouraged

[insert appropriate feeling here]

because:

Here is my solution to this bullshit:

Day 7
Week 12

A DIRTY WORD

"Well, for starters, I'm a millionaire. I'm also a mom with three young kids, a bonus daughter, and a loving husband, and I'm the employer of over a dozen people."
~Rachel Rodgers

Today's goals...

Habit	Goals	Outcomes
Sleep		
Water		
Food		
Fitness		
Steps		
Stress		
Habit: ____________		
Habit: ____________		
Habit: ____________		

A MOMENT OF GRATITUDE

Well, for starters, I'm a

____

[insert a noun that lets people know you are badass and fierce].
I'm also a mom with

____

[insert number] young/teen/adult children,

____

a [insert occupation], and I make a difference in the world by

____

[insert your response]. I'm grateful.

Daily Shit: Reflections about Today's Goals and Outcomes

I'm the **SHIT** because:

I am proud of this because:

This is how I am going to build on that:

Today's **BULLSHIT** is this:

I feel frustrated, disappointed, angry, discouraged

[insert appropriate feeling here]

because:

Here is my solution to this bullshit:

THE WEEKLY TEA ... SPILL IT

What are you most proud of this week?

What challenged you this week?

What lessons will you take with you into next week?

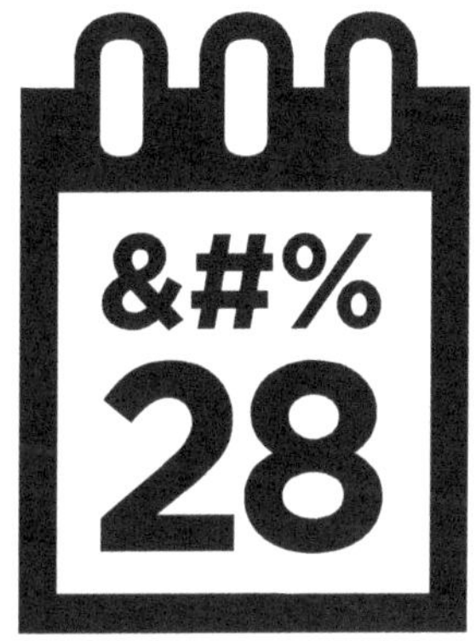

Monthly Shit

You made it through 28 days!
Let's check in using the self-confidence and
self-value exercises that follow.

Self-Value Tank

At the top of each tank, please write a value that you have worked to honor over the past four weeks. For example, you may indicate prayer, good sleep hygiene or healthy touch. Next, indicate how much energy you've put into that value by coloring or shading in the corresponding amount of "gas" you've poured into that particular tank.

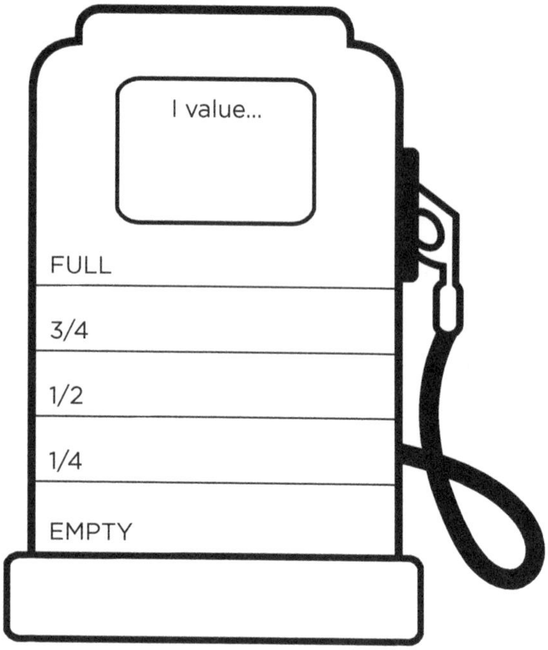

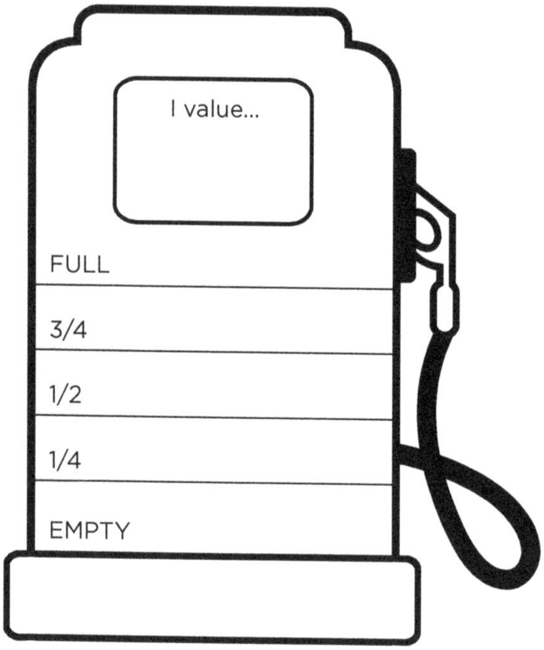

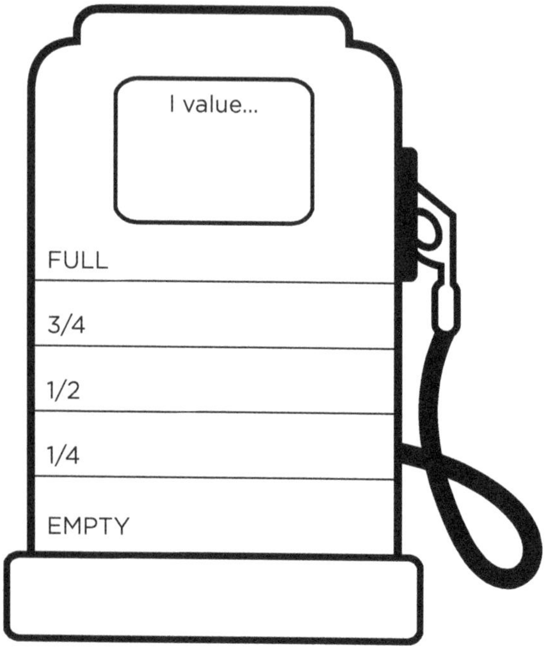

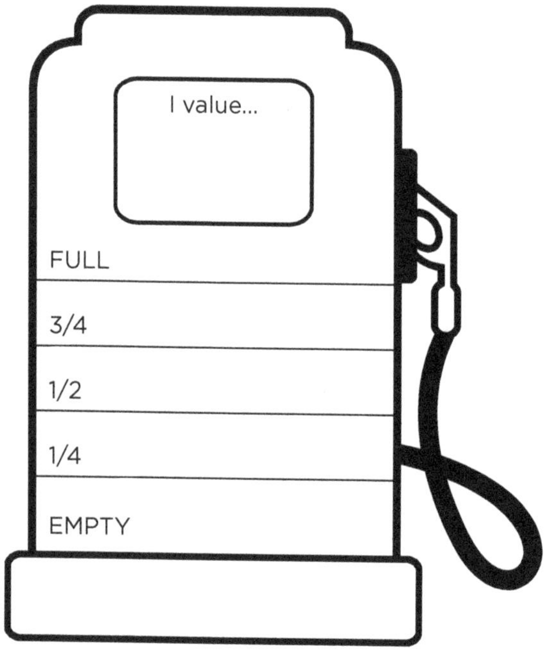

Self-Value Tank Reflection

Self-Confidence Scale

At the end of every month, you will be asked to fill in the layers based on how you are feeling that day and the level of trust have in your ability to overcome your current challenges.

Do you trust yourself to meet your health and wellness goals?

Do you feel that you can meet your health and wellness goals?

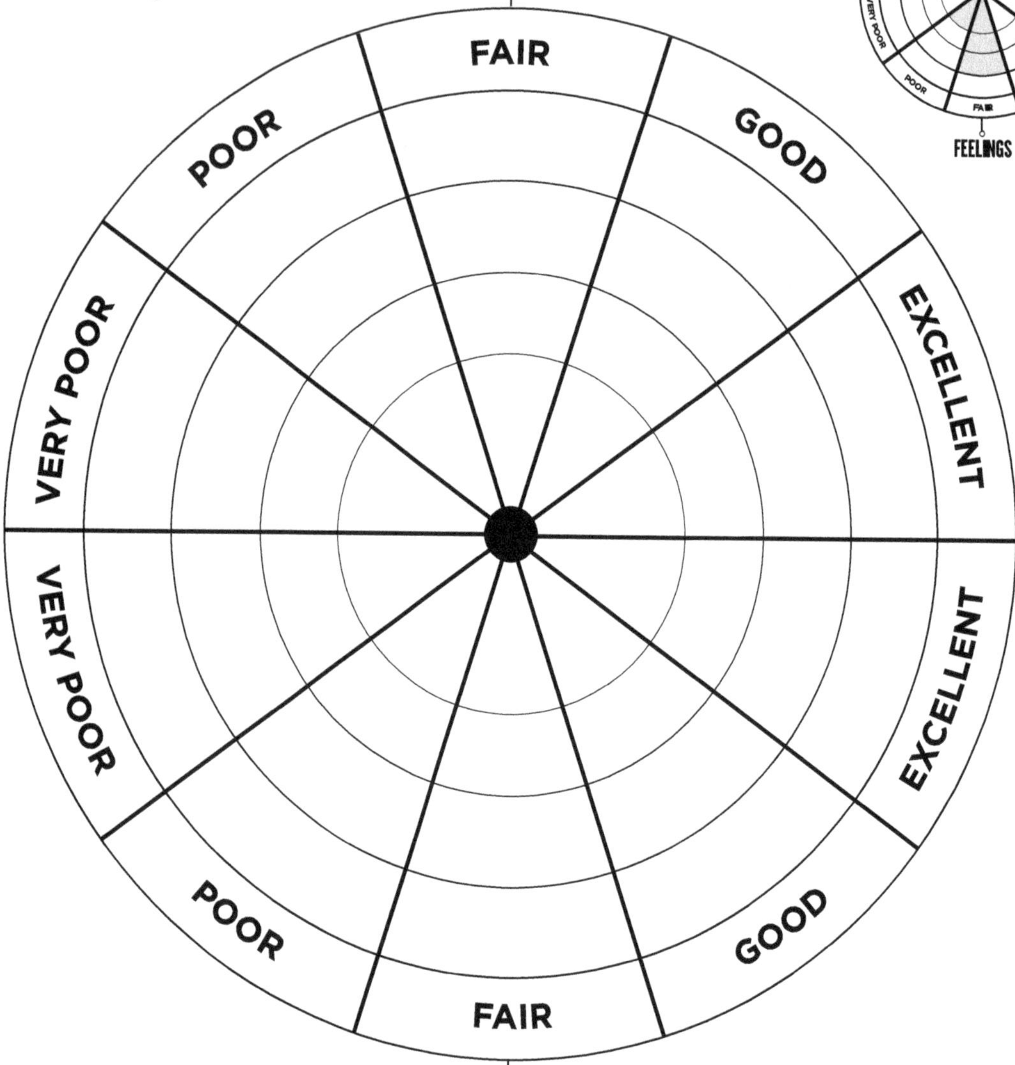

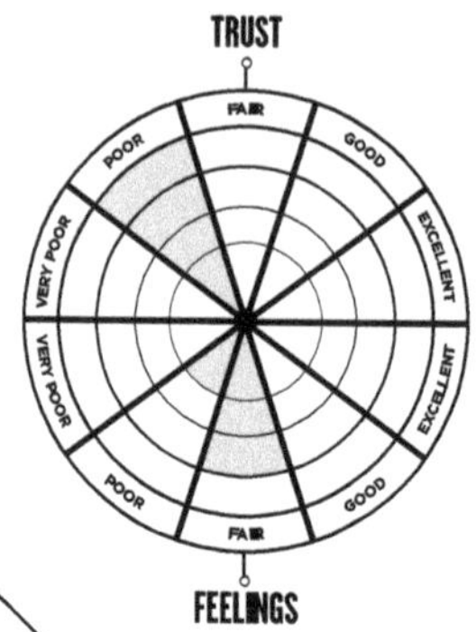

Self-Confidence Scale Reflection

12-Week Summary

12w You know you are fierce! Completing your 12-week plan is just one more example of your boss ways. You owned your health and wellness goals over these past weeks. In the space below, please reflect on anything from the emotions you felt, goals you accomplished, mindsets you faced to the spiritual battles you've overcome over these last three months. You may want to write about lessons you've learned and discoveries you've made about yourself. You may not want to reflect on any of these at all. Instead, you may want to focus strictly on numbers—the amount of steps you took, pounds you lost, calories you burned, number of days you met your sleep goals. Or you may want to write about your story and your numbers. Use this space in ways that best serve you as you close out this part of your journey and prepare for the next phase.

Measurements

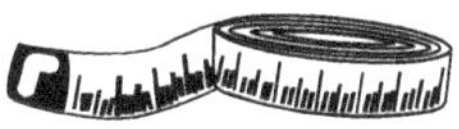

In wealth, it's crucial to keep track of your numbers. The same holds true in health. Knowing your measurements is a way to track progress. The scale gives you one piece of information. But that information is not always complete. Measurements can help you balance the books. It can also give you a sense of how your workouts are transforming your body over time.

But where to begin? Start by gathering the right "tools." At the very least, you will need a flexible, inelastic tape measure. Consider a cloth one. You will also need a full-length mirror to increase the likelihood of accurate measurements. (If you are really fancy, buy a body fat calculator to determine your body fat percentage. But this journal does not use that measurement method, so it will not be covered here.)

What will you measure? As you progress on your health and wellness journey, your body composition is likely to change. For this reason, you must measure more than one part of your body to get a snapshot of any changes that have occurred. It is suggested that you measure the following parts of your body:

- Left and right upper arm
- Chest
- Waist
- Hips
- Left and right thigh

How do you measure each suggested part? Consistency is very important. Be consistent about the time of day that you measure your body. A "Verywell Fit" article offers this bit of advice: "It's a great idea to take your measurements first thing in the morning before eating or drinking anything. Every time you retake your measurements, take them at the same time, and under the same circumstances, so you can trust the results."[5] With regard to timing, experts agree that you should not measure yourself daily, with suggestions varying from every week to every four weeks. In this journal, we are recommending that you measure yourself every four weeks.

For those interested in keeping this process simple, here are some basic rules of thumb. First, measure the smallest circumference of your waist but the largest circumference of your hips, thighs, arms, and chest. Second, for your stomach, find the midpoint between your belly button and breast bone to measure your waist circumference. Third, for your hips, wrap the tape around your body at the widest point between your butt and hips. These three tips taken from a Livestrong.com article may be easier to remember than the more detailed suggestions that come next.

Some of you may be looking for a process that feels "more precise." In that case, please consider these suggestions offered by Covet's lead fitness instructor, Gretchen Treiber Girard:

5 https://www.verywellfit.com/how-to-take-your-body-measurements-1231126

Girth Measurements

When most of us talk about our desire to lose weight, we want to lose fat. Sometimes you can step on the scale and see that your weight loss has slowed or even stopped. The number frustratingly doesn't budge, but you are in fact losing fat as you notice your clothes feeling a little looser, your movements coming a little easier. You can still lose fat and gain lean body mass. For this reason, one of the best ways to measure success with a fat loss journey is to do girth measurements—measure the circumference of certain anatomical landmarks.

When you are taking measurements, it is important to be as accurate as possible. To ensure you have a consistent method for measuring, use the exact same landmarks and use a pen to mark the skin where the tape measure will go, perhaps take a picture of those markings, and have someone else—preferably the same person—do the measurements for you. Also, be sure the measuring tape is always snug enough to lay flat against the skin but not tight enough to press into the skin.

Chest: To take the chest measurement, simply place one end of the tape measure around the fullest part of the chest then wrap under the armpits. It should also be over the shoulder blades and back-to-front for an accurate reading.

Upper Arm, R & L: Stand tall with arms hanging freely and hands facing the body. Measure the middle of the area between the elbow and the tip of the shoulder.

Waist: Stand tall with arms hanging freely, feet together, and abdomen relaxed (no sucking in!;). Measure the narrowest part of the torso, above the belly button and below the ribs.

Hips/Buttocks: Stand tall with feet together, and measure the area around the maximal circumference of the buttocks, usually just below the hip bones.

Upper Thigh, R & L: Stand tall with legs slightly apart, and measure the widest point between the groin and the knee; this is usually just below the lowest part of the buttocks (aka the "shelf")

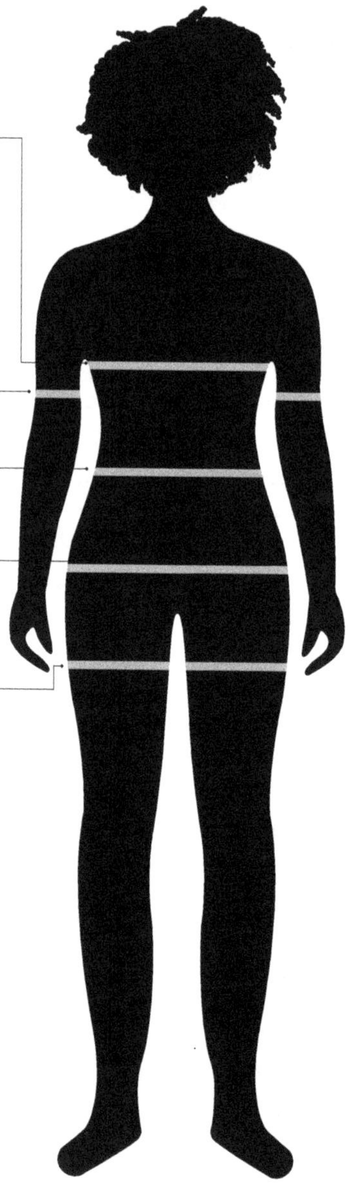

NOTES:

- "Standing tall" means standing in neutral spine with shoulders stacked—ears over shoulders over hips, hips over ankles, and shoulders pulled down and back.
- The directions are written as if the measurer is the self being measured, even though the recommended process of measuring is to have someone else do the measuring.

YOUR MEASUREMENTS

Record your starting measurements here. Take the measurements once a week. Pick a day of week and measure yourself at the same time of that day. Keep in mind, sometimes the scale does not yield the results, but measurements do.

WEEK:

Arm	Chest	Waist	Hip	Leg

WEEK:

Arm	Chest	Waist	Hip	Leg

WEEK:

Arm	Chest	Waist	Hip	Leg

WEEK:

Arm	Chest	Waist	Hip	Leg

WEEK:

Arm	Chest	Waist	Hip	Leg

WEEK:

Arm	Chest	Waist	Hip	Leg

WEEK:

Arm	Chest	Waist	Hip	Leg

WEEK:

Arm	Chest	Waist	Hip	Leg

WEEK:

Arm	Chest	Waist	Hip	Leg

WEEK:

Arm	Chest	Waist	Hip	Leg

WEEK:

Arm	Chest	Waist	Hip	Leg

WEEK:

Arm	Chest	Waist	Hip	Leg

CPSIA information can be obtained
at www.ICGtesting.com
Printed in the USA
BVHW061448210322
631558BV00003B/5

9 781955 656153